Hypothyroidism in Childhood and Adulthood

A personal perspective and scientific standpoint

Hypothyroidism in Childhood and Adulthood

A personal perspective and scientific standpoint

By C Phillips BSc (Hons) and D Roach BSc (Hons)

First published by Nottingham University Press

This reissued original edition published 2023 by 5m Books Ltd www.5mbooks.com

British Library Cataloguing in Publication Data
Hypothyroidism in Childhood and Adulthood

ISBN   9781789182866

Disclaimer

Every reasonable effort has been made to ensure that the material in this book is true, correct, complete and appropriate at the time of writing. Nevertheless the publishers, the editors and the authors do not accept responsibility for any omission or error, or for any injury, damage, loss or financial consequences arising from the use of the book.

Medical Disclaimer

In this book, the authors have described their experiences of hypothyroidism during childhood and adulthood from a personal perspective and a scientific standpoint, in order to highlight difficulties that they have experienced with regard to the diagnosis, monitoring and treatment of hypothyroidism. The information contained in this book relates to the individual experiences of the authors and should not be used to diagnose disease or prescribe medicine and the publisher and authors and anyone involved in the production of this book assume no responsibility for such action. Anyone requiring diagnosis, monitoring or treatment should always consult a qualified medical doctor on an individual basis. This is *not* a medical book.

Typeset by Nottingham University Press, Nottingham

EU GPSR Authorised Representative
LOGOS EUROPE, 9 rue Nicolas Poussin, 17000, LA ROCHELLE, France
E-mail: Contact@logoseurope.eu

Front cover illustration by CFCF: https://commons.wikimedia.org/wiki/File:Posterior_thyroid.jpg#/media/File:Posterior_thyroid.jpg

ABOUT THE AUTHORS

C Phillips and D Roach are identical twin sisters who have both suffered from hypothyroidism during childhood and again during adulthood (due to a reduction in their treatment). They have therefore been able to describe experiences of hypothyroidism from a personal perspective. As they are both science graduates, they were also able to document their experiences from a scientific standpoint.

ACKNOWLEDGEMENTS

We are grateful to our family for their love and support during our illness and their encouragement during the preparation of this book.

Heartfelt thanks must go to J Cameron MBA for her help in the preparation of this book and D Phillips BSc MSc for his invaluable IT skills.

We are extremely grateful to the specialist paediatrician who diagnosed our childhood hypothyroidism and monitored our treatment throughout childhood. Sadly this excellent doctor died during 2004.

In addition, we would like to thank the friend who urged us to revisit our NHS GP immediately as emergency cases and request repeat blood tests, which prompted a partial increase in our thyroxine (T4) dose in 2001.

We would like to convey our sincere thanks to our private doctor for correcting the under-treatment of our hypothyroidism during adulthood and helping us towards recovery. In addition, we would like to thank the NHS endocrinologists and NHS GPs who have enabled us to obtain our current treatment via the NHS.

Finally we wish to thank all those individuals and groups who have provided encouragement and support during the production of this book.

To our family and friends with love

CONTENTS

GLOSSARY

DXA scan
This is used to measure the density of bone so that it can be classified as normal, osteopenic or osteoporotic.

Endocrine system
This is comprised of glands, which secrete chemical substances known as hormones, which have various effects on different parts of the body.

Euthyroid
In the euthyroid state, the thyroid gland produces sufficient thyroid hormones.

Hyperthyroidism
The thyroid gland produces surplus thyroid hormones.

Hypothyroidism
The thyroid gland produces insufficient thyroid hormones.

National Health Service (NHS)
In the United Kingdom (UK) the National Health Service (NHS) was established in 1948 so that the government could provide health care in the UK, funded through National Insurance contributions from citizens of the UK.

Osteopenia
This is when the bone density is below normal but above osteoporotic. Bone tissue is continually being broken down and replaced (a higher rate of bone breakdown increases the risk of osteoporosis).

Osteoporosis
This is when the bone density is below normal and below osteopenic, thus increasing the risk of bone fractures.

Thyroid
This is a gland in the neck that secretes the thyroid hormones.

Thyroid hormones
Thyroxine (T4) and **tri-iodothyronine (T3)** are two of the thyroid hormones secreted by the thyroid gland and are needed for metabolism, energy production, growth and development. **Di-iodothyronine (T2)** and **mono-iodothyronine (T1)** are also produced by the thyroid gland.

The thyroid hormone treatments referred to in this book, include **thyroxine (T4)**, **tri-iodothyronine (T3)** and **natural desiccated thyroid (NDT)** treatment (porcine derived).

The generic name for the thyroxine (T4) prescribed for us was 'thyroxine tablets BP', which contain synthetic thyroxine sodium. The generic name for the tri-iodothyronine (T3) prescribed for us was 'liothyronine sodium BP' which contains synthetic tri-iodothyronine sodium. BP is the abbreviation for British Pharmacopoeia.

The **NDT treatment** (porcine derived) prescribed for us, was Armour™ Thyroid (thyroid tablets, USP). Armour™ Thyroid is copyright© 2005 Forest Pharmaceuticals, Inc. and USP is the abbreviation for United States Pharmacopoeia.

Thyroid stimulating hormone (TSH)
This hormone is produced by the pituitary gland and stimulates the thyroid gland to produce thyroid hormones. If the thyroid gland produces insufficient thyroid hormone, TSH production is normally stimulated whilst, if the thyroid gland produces excessive thyroid hormone, TSH production is normally suppressed.

Urine deoxypyridinoline (Dpd) levels
Deoxypyridinoline (Dpd) is one of the bone breakdown products present in the urine. Higher urine Dpd levels indicate a higher rate of bone breakdown.

Urine N-telopeptide (NTx) levels
N-telopeptide (NTx) is one of the bone breakdown products present in urine. Higher urine NTx levels indicate a higher rate of bone breakdown.

Waking temperature
Dr Broda Barnes carried out research into the correlation between hypothyroidism and a subnormal body temperature on waking.

INTRODUCTION

By C Phillips BSc and D Roach BSc

We are identical twin sisters who developed a thyroid failure during childhood, one after the other. We were fortunate that the paediatrician to whom we were referred made an accurate diagnosis of hypothyroidism, resulting in appropriate treatment of our condition. We were thus able to regain our health and develop normally. We were advised that we would need prescriptions for daily thyroid treatment for the rest of our lives.

As adults, we were satisfied with the thyroxine (T4) dose that we had taken since childhood because it relieved all of our physical symptoms of hypothyroidism. However during adulthood, National Health Service (NHS) concerns over the possibility of a link between a suppressed thyroid stimulating hormone (TSH) level and risk of premature osteoporosis led to the reduction of the thyroxine dose, that we had taken since childhood. DXA hip scans were taken and the results are shown in appendices 1 to 4.

However, we decided to keep detailed records in order to evaluate reductions in our thyroxine dose. We kept records of blood test results (see appendix 5 for blood test results). We kept records of urine N-telopeptide (NTx) levels (see appendix 6 for urine N-telopeptide (NTx) levels). We also kept a daily diary. In this way, we hoped that we would soon be treated with the best thyroxine dose for both our wellbeing and our bone health.

During changes to our thyroxine dose carried out by NHS doctors, we experienced difficulties that they had not anticipated (due to under-treatment of our hypothyroidism) and kept records that could not be collected deliberately via an academic research study because such a study would be unethical and life threatening. Therefore, we felt a duty to share our information with researchers in this field. In our case, there was not a consistent correlation between our blood test results and our symptoms of hypothyroidism.

During our recovery from under-treated hypothyroidism, we had the opportunity to experience treatment with thyroxine, tri-iodothyronine (T3) and natural desiccated thyroid (NDT) treatment (porcine derived) and to compare their efficacy in our situation. In this book, we have documented our search in consultation with all the doctors who treated us, for the thyroid treatment best suited to our individual needs. This book is based upon our personal experiences during our search for wellness. We have written from a personal perspective in part 1 and a scientific standpoint in part 2.

'Time wasted is existence, used is life'

Edward Young

PART 1

EXPERIENCES OF HYPOTHYROIDISM FROM A PERSONAL PERSPECTIVE

Preface to Part 1

In part 1, identical twin sisters (D Roach and C Phillips) have outlined their experiences of hypothyroidism in both childhood and adulthood from a personal perspective. They have tried to convey the impact of hypothyroidism on their daily lives and the emotional, practical and financial implications of this condition.

In chapter 1, D Roach has written about the devastating effects of hypothyroidism in childhood from a personal perspective. In addition, D Roach has detailed the development of symptoms of hypothyroidism in adulthood following the reduction in her thyroxine (T4) treatment.

In chapter 2, C Phillips has described hypothyroidism in childhood from her personal perspective. Prior to experiencing the condition herself, C Phillips witnessed the detrimental effects of hypothyroidism on her identical twin sister's health. C Phillips has recounted the reality of under treated hypothyroidism during adulthood, which had a debilitating effect on her health.

CHAPTER 1

MARCH 1969 –SEPTEMBER 2004

HYPOTHYROIDISM FROM A PERSONAL PERSPECTIVE

By D Roach

As an identical twin, my earliest memories of childhood were of always having my twin sister's company and spending hours playing energetic games with each other and with friends. However, during my time at junior school I felt as if my energy was ebbing away and I no longer wanted to play in the playground. My family would comment that my sister's shoes were always scuffed whilst mine remained shiny and as good as new. During break times, I sat on the sidelines and watched the other children race around. Returning to the classroom was an immense effort and if I had to climb stairs, I would become out of breath even though I stopped to rest on each step. I could not walk at normal speeds but as a child, I accepted this without question.

As for schoolwork, my mind started to go blank when asked questions during lessons and it became difficult to concentrate. The above deterioration in my wellbeing was extremely gradual and insidious. However, because I had an identical twin sister, the contrast between our development became increasingly obvious with time. My twin sister grew taller than I, whilst my growth was stunted and people who did not know us assumed that I was a younger sister rather than an identical twin. In fact I was a few minutes older than my twin sister.

My face was puffy and I also seemed to put on weight despite sticking to low calorie diets recommended by my general practitioners (GPs). My face became pale despite taking the iron supplements that were prescribed for me. My scalp was dry and my hair started falling out despite the use of recommended shampoos.

My parents were very concerned about me and they knew that I should really be progressing like my sister. After going back and forth to the doctor's surgery over a couple of years, I was eventually seen by a specialist paediatrician, who promptly diagnosed me with hypothyroidism and treated me with thyroxine (T4) tablets. I have always been extremely thankful to that doctor who treated me when I was a child and I now have no doubt that he saved my life. My recovery proved to be remarkable and over time, I lost weight, regained my energy, increased in height and began to develop normally for my age. Eventually, I also managed to catch up with my academic work.

During this time, I was honoured to be able to contribute to university medical lectures by providing photographs taken before and after commencement of my thyroxine treatment, with my sister alongside me for the purposes of comparison. Our family hoped that these photographs would help new doctors to make an early diagnosis of childhood hypothyroidism. This gave us an opportunity to provide incontrovertible scientific evidence (in the form of official photographs for medical purposes) which clearly illustrated the devastation that untreated hypothyroidism can cause during childhood. These photographs are shown in part 2 of this book.

I was monitored carefully by my paediatrician throughout my childhood, so I never had to worry about my thyroid condition. When my twin sister also developed hypothyroidism during childhood (a few years after my diagnosis), she was diagnosed, treated and monitored by the same specialist as myself. Eventually, we again became more alike in appearance and academic ability. People again became confused about which twin was which (as had happened prior to our childhood hypothyroidism). We both went on to successfully complete a science degree at university.

As an adult, I never dwelt on the fact that I'd had a thyroid failure during childhood. As far as I was concerned, as long as I continued to take my tablets I was at no disadvantage to anyone else. I found employment and eventually I got married.

In adulthood I continued to take the same thyroxine treatment as I had taken since childhood. Since childhood, my sister and I had both taken thyroxine with a brand name but some time during our mid-twenties, we both had our treatment changed to generic thyroxine.

One disadvantage of hypothyroidism was having the occasional blood test. One such blood test to monitor my treatment led to my daily thyroxine dose being slightly lowered in the Summer of 1999. I felt concerned that I was developing symptoms of under treated hypothyroidism. I felt cold and unwell. I could not take a shower without crouching and shivering. However, my thyroxine dose was returned to its original level in Spring 2000 on my request. Even though my symptoms improved when my dose was returned to the original level, I was informed that it was clinically impossible for my symptoms to have been caused by the dose reduction because my thyroid stimulating hormone (TSH) level had remained suppressed. Nevertheless, after a relatively short reduction in my treatment, on returning to my original thyroxine dosage, my recovery was relatively smooth.

NHS doctors were worried in case there was any link between suppressed TSH levels and reduced bone density and I was put on waiting lists for bone scans (and so was my sister). Following bone scans which showed that our hip bones were thinner than expected, my sister and I were warned by NHS doctors that we needed to reduce our thyroxine dose until our TSH levels were 'normal'. In light of my previous dose reduction, we both felt deeply concerned about this news.

This was a nightmarish situation. I did not want to reduce my thyroxine dose again if it meant suffering symptoms of hypothyroidism but I could not remain on the same thyroxine dose if NHS doctors were anxious that I was at risk of imminent premature osteoporosis. After such warnings, I was of course concerned about getting premature osteoporosis but I could not be certain that lowering my thyroxine dose was the answer.

My sister and I sat in a café and discussed our dilemma whilst scribbling notes on a serviette. We were not aware of ever having experienced symptoms of over treatment of our thyroid failure during adulthood. Since our daily thyroxine dose was to be lowered, we decided that it was important for us to monitor our wellbeing in daily diaries so that our dosage could be reviewed if any decline in our wellbeing occurred. We would also look into ways of monitoring our bone health. We hoped that the best thyroxine dose for both our wellbeing and our bone health would soon be found.

In March 2001, I saw my NHS GP and lowered my daily thyroxine dose by a quarter. One of my first observations was that I felt as if there wasn't enough oxygen in the air and I therefore had to breathe more deeply. I began experiencing pins and needles in my hands. Subsequently I began feeling very tired. My appetite decreased. My sleep requirements increased. I had always walked everywhere but noted that it took me longer to walk short distances. I found exercising a struggle. I started to feel fuzzy headed, heavy and exhausted. I noticed that I felt cold in work when no one else did and that I had cold hands. I experienced an aching chest.

Blood test results appeared to be influential with regard to decisions about the level of thyroxine treatment that I should take. Although I reported my symptoms to my GP surgery, further blood test results led to my thyroxine dose being halved compared to what I had originally been taking. Despite adequate sleep, I still felt very tired throughout the day. I noted that my hands ached whilst making a cup of tea, putting clothes away and other light tasks. My symptoms were ongoing.

I had yet another blood test and by this time, I had begun to encounter real difficulties in the work place because of my aching hands and other symptoms and by June 2001, I was no longer able to work. I visited my GP again but was informed that my body would soon 'adjust' to my reduced treatment and I would be able to return to work. I wished I knew how long the 'adjustment' would last.

In addition to ongoing symptoms already described, I also noted that I had headaches. I had a further blood test. In my diary I observed that more of my hair seemed to be falling out than usual. Something was not right but I hoped that I would soon improve as predicted by my GP. One night I described in my diary how I had woken up in the early hours with severely aching muscles throughout my body, chest ache, headache and terrible hand/ forearm pain. Writing in my diary was painful. It was painful to walk.

I felt as if I was muddling up my words. I found that I fell asleep during the daytime. I noted that my hands ached when I tried to carry out simple every day tasks such as writing some birthday cards or peeling fruit. I felt as if I was less able to think in a clear and focused way and found everything a ridiculous effort. One weekend after a short walk I went to bed at 5pm and slept for 15 hours and another 3 hours during the following day. I found that I had to wear bigger sizes and baggy outfits because I couldn't fit into my usual clothes.

Despite everything, I continued to record my symptoms in a daily diary as previously planned. I described for example, how I had woken up with painful hands in the middle of the night, crying out in pain.

Tasks such as bathing and dressing were difficult because of drowsiness and hand pains. After some time, I had insufficient strength to even spray deodorant. I was feeling exhausted despite continual rest or sleep. I felt less talkative. In addition to symptoms described I also noted having aching hips.

My hand pains worsened and in desperation I sought more advice from the NHS. I did not feel that I was able to adequately convey the severity of my symptoms to my doctors. Perhaps the lowering of the thyroxine dose was necessary to prevent premature osteoporosis. Perhaps I would adjust to the half dose soon. However I was concerned about my increasing symptoms.

I continued to consult my GP. I had so many symptoms that I worried in case I was dismissed as a hypochondriac. I wore supports on my forearms but I still suffered hand pain that reduced me to tears. I was feeling too exhausted to do normal activities. Intermittent chest pains were very disconcerting. Next I started having a sick/ queasy sensation which restricted activity even further. I consulted another GP. I began having back pain.

I was only aware of thinking approximately half a dozen thoughts during the day. I felt as if I had slipped into some sort of stupor. I started having tinnitus, earache and balance problems. Although I felt as if someone had drugged me with pills to make me sleep, I was still concerned at the parallel symptoms that my sister was experiencing and my sister was concerned at the symptoms that I was experiencing. Therefore my sister and I revisited our GP to request an urgent review of our thyroxine dose and a further blood test in view of our increasing symptoms.

I described in my diary how I was feeling really ill as if I was under attack from inside. Then at last I was contacted by my GP. My TSH had risen well above normal showing that I did need a higher thyroxine dose. Now that my blood tests confirmed what I had been saying, I had to go to my surgery immediately and increase my thyroxine dose to three-quarters of what it had been originally.

At this point I felt as if I was very travel sick, especially when I moved my head. I was unable to do housework, shop, do normal tasks, cook or look after myself. I noted having visual disturbances (occasionally I saw a black blob on the periphery of my vision that I initially mistook to be a spider). I also had spinal pain and I worried that this was due to the onset of premature osteoporosis after all the concerns that NHS doctors had expressed. In addition I was often in tears because of the pain all over my body.

On top of everything else, I had stabbing pains in the eyes. I also had pains in the jaw. I paid privately to see a NHS endocrinologist who was hopeful that the partial increase in my dose would help me to regain my health. I felt really low by that time. I also experienced pain at the base of my spine. I was taken on a short car journey and then I retched into hankies.

I followed the advice of the NHS endocrinologist that I had seen and had further blood tests. Due to nausea and balance problems and other symptoms, I was housebound. I felt as if I was trapped on a ship sailing rough seas. Each day I hoped that the next day would be better. The nausea caused me to make retching noises. I had always been very hard working but now I was rendered functionless and the whole experience was very frightening. My balance problems led to countless falls in the house.

I was able to go to a shop if I held onto someone but if I let go I often lost my balance and fell. It crossed my mind that strangers in shops would think that I was drunk or drugged or weird. If I was standing up and someone asked me a question, all my concentration would be diverted to answering their question rather than standing up and it was not unusual for me to lose my balance at this point and to fall over.

Seven weeks after increasing my thyroxine dose back to three quarters of its original level, I had pinching chest pains that lasted for a couple of hours. This was reported to my GP. I saw another NHS specialist in relation to my hand pains and was put on another long waiting list.

Very small improvements occurred but I was still suffering from many symptoms. I saw another NHS endocrinologist. I saw my GP. I had another blood test. I had another bone scan. After all that the NHS doctors had said, I was very worried about the results of the bone scan. The results were similar to the first scan that I had been given. I continued to keep a diary. Another NHS specialist that I saw was very helpful and assured me that I did not need annual bone scans and did not need to have another one until I was menopausal.

My symptoms were ongoing and I continued to have balance problems and countless falls. As mentioned my dose had been increased slightly but something still felt very wrong. I was then told that on this dose my blood tests were 'normal'. It was deeply worrying that symptoms and blood test results told a very different story. My exhaustion was indescribable, in the morning I would lie on the settee and in the afternoon I would still be lying down in the same position. I would often have to go to bed during early evening.

Any activity was painstakingly slow and difficult but I sent letters to various places and NHS doctors for advice. I had put my trust in the NHS and had waited patiently for each GP or specialist consultation, hoping desperately that the next consultation would result in an urgent review of my treatment and when this did not happen, I was devastated. After nearly a year and a half of ill health I was given the impression that there was no alternative to my ongoing symptoms of hypothyroidism due to my risk of premature osteoporosis.

My mother took my twin sister and myself to see our GP and requested that we be referred to a private doctor who had sent helpful replies to our letters. Following our referral to this private doctor in September 2002, our thyroxine dose was returned to what it had been all along. I soon noticed feeling a little warmer. Previously it would not be unusual for me to be wrapped in layers of clothes underneath a blanket even when the weather was fine (despite leaving the central heating on all day). My appetite increased suddenly and I demolished the mismatched contents of the fridge during one meal but after that my appetite came back to normal. My head started to feel less fuzzy. My energy was still very low and I often rested on the settee all day.

I started to experience relief from back pain and coccyx or lower back pain. I noticed becoming more talkative. I was relieved when I began to have days without the frightening experience of intermittent chest ache. I began to have some relief from nausea, retching and tinnitus. Eventually, the active thyroid hormone tri-iodothyronine (T3) was included in my treatment but any changes to my thyroid treatment had to be made very gradually.

I had only ever taken one of the thyroid hormones i.e. synthetic thyroxine and was very apprehensive about trying synthetic T3 for the first time. I broke one little tablet into 4 pieces and planned to take one quarter of a tablet only on the first day. Less than half an hour after taking T3, I had temporary relief from my balance problems until the effects of the T3 faded. Although my balance problems would come back abruptly, it was good to have some brief relief from balance problems during the day.

My colour perception improved. The world seemed sharper and brighter as if my colour perception had dulled without me realizing. My perception of the world was unexpectedly altered as if I had removed dark tinted sunglasses or turned up the brightness switch on the television.

After being housebound for a prolonged period, I risked going for very short walks during the temporary improvements in my balance. However I shouldn't really have done this because my balance was unreliable and my balance problems would suddenly return without warning. Then I would have to phone someone to help me make the short walk home.

After consultation with my private doctor, the ratio of T3 was very gradually increased. I continued to have blood tests. I gradually improved so that I was experiencing relief from some of the symptoms that I'd been having prior to seeing my private doctor.

I still had to be relatively restful as I did not have the energy or stamina to do much. The T3 could get used up quickly and symptoms would return abruptly. If I was restful for a few days, I could then have just enough energy to go out with family but for the following few days, my energy was utterly drained and I would have to be extremely restful again. Frustratingly brief activity would be curtailed by energy depletion and worsening symptoms. I still had problems with my hands, sometimes they would be painful during hand usage and sometimes later on and this restricted how much I could do.

I had a further consultation with my private doctor. My T3 dose was gradually increased and my thyroxine dose was lowered. At this time I had experienced daily symptoms of hypothyroidism for over 2 years (excluding the previous time period 2 years prior to that during which my thyroxine dose had been lowered and raised again).

Unlike the year 2000, my recovery from a longer more drastic dose reduction was not at all quick or smooth. Getting over severe/ longstanding under treatment of hypothyroidism was difficult and slow. Having my thyroid treatment partially withdrawn was a devastating experience and was followed by loss of health, work, marriage and home with obvious practical, financial and emotional implications. Thankfully I had found an excellent doctor who was helping me to recover. In addition I was grateful for the loving support of family and friends.

Further increases in my T3 dose and decreases in my thyroxine dose were made. My puffiness disappeared but I continued to have exhaustion, pain in my hands and balance problems. My level of activity gradually increased but my stamina was still extremely low. It was a bit like having batteries which kept needing to be recharged all the time.

I had further blood tests and went to see my private doctor again. Due to my remaining symptoms and lack of stamina, my T3 treatment was gradually reduced and simultaneously replaced with natural desiccated thyroid (NDT) treatment (porcine derived). Eventually, I was treated with NDT treatment (porcine derived) only and I was delighted to be making further progress in my recovery. Whenever any alterations in my thyroid treatment occurred, I gradually altered the timing and spacing of my tablet taking to suit my individual needs.

Words could not adequately describe my gratitude towards my private doctor for helping me with my ongoing recovery from under treated hypothyroidism. I knew that taking NDT treatment (porcine derived) would remain essential for my continuing progress and it was a wonderful experience to be on the road to recovery.

CHAPTER 2

MARCH 1969 – SEPTEMBER 2004

HYPOTHYROIDISM FROM A PERSONAL PERSPECTIVE

By C Phillips

I know differently now, but when I was a child, the world had seemed a fair place, my sister and I (being identical twins) received exactly the same treatment from those around us. We wore the same or similar clothes and were chosen for the same roles in the school Christmas concert.

Then, suddenly the world stopped being fair, my sister started to have lower marks than me at school. I was growing but my sister remained shorter than myself and started to become extremely puffy. My sister was taken back and forth to the GP in a desperate attempt to obtain treatment for her problems. However low calorie diets and iron tablets recommended by GPs did not result in any improvement.

At playtime, my sister would spend the entire break sitting on the wall and struggled to get up the school steps, taking one step at a time and stopping on each step. Just as my sister couldn't muster the energy to run and play, I couldn't prevent myself from doing so.

Then worst of all, I found out that my sister was being demoted to a different class. At that age, I was incredulous at the injustice of this event. I remember my mother having a private chat with me, to share her concerns about the future. Although I was developing normally, my mother feared that my twin sister might never be able to regain normal development (mental and physical).

Eventually the GPs agreed to let my sister see a specialist paediatrician who diagnosed my sister with a thyroid failure and treated her with thyroxine (T4). As my sister recovered, we would do our separate homework but my sister insisted on doing extra homework to catch up with me until she was eventually promoted to the same class as me again. When we were in different classes, I remember making a cardboard puppet in class and remember my mother rushing out to buy cardboard and string so that my sister could make a cardboard puppet in the house. All my family did their best to ensure that my sister didn't miss out as a result of her illness.

When I started to develop hypothyroidism, I didn't question my reduced energy, breathlessness and weight gain. Neither did I complain. I accepted that I was just a 'dawdler' and that I had 'puppy fat'. Perhaps my passive acceptance was in itself a symptom.

Fortunately, my mother requested a blood test and I was diagnosed with hypothyroidism and started on thyroxine treatment. We moved house and changed to a different school. The specialist paediatrician who had diagnosed and treated my sister's hypothyroidism treated my hypothyroidism also. He continued to see us for a six monthly check up throughout our childhood and took great care in ensuring that we remained symptom free.

We took our thyroxine tablets in the same way as someone might take vitamin tablets, with no expectation that our hypothyroidism would ever return. As adults, our hypothyroidism was no longer something we talked about or even thought about very often. I went to university and gained a 2.1 Bachelor of Science degree with Honours, found employment and later got married.

Following a blood test, my sister was asked to reduce her daily thyroxine dose. Unfortunately, my sister's health subsequently declined until my sister's dose was eventually increased again to its previous level (on my sister's request) and her health subsequently improved. However, this was not the end of the matter, the doctors were concerned that there could be a link between a suppressed TSH level and reduced bone density and she was given a wrist scan. This demonstrated osteopenia and she was put on a waiting list for a hip scan.

Out of concern, I was also sent for a wrist scan which came out normal but I asked to have a hip scan too.

Both our hip scans showed osteopenia and due to our suppressed TSH levels, we were both told to reduce our daily dose of thyroxine until our TSH levels normalised.

There was talk of osteopenia leading to imminent premature osteoporosis and osteoporosis leading to hip fracture and the risks associated with this. I realised that we had no choice but to reduce our thyroxine dose in March 2001 to three-quarters of its original level but hoped that we would not suffer the same problems that my sister had suffered when her dose had been reduced previously.

Sitting in a café discussing the matter, we felt as though we had no option but to try reducing our dose but should keep such detailed records that if we did have a problem, we could go back to the doctors immediately.

Shortly after reducing my dose to three-quarters of its original level, I started to develop symptoms. I was informed that most of my symptoms were due to my need for adjustment to my new dose and should go soon and if they didn't go, they weren't related to the hypothyroidism.

Following a blood test, my dose was further reduced to half its original level. I deteriorated further and was soon unable to continue working and made several visits to the GP but I was informed repeatedly that most of my symptoms were due to the need for adjustment to my new dose.

I felt troubled but without the benefit of being able to see into the future, I had no way of knowing that my symptoms wouldn't go soon and I was also worried about the threat of premature osteoporosis. In addition, two consecutive blood test results had satisfied the doctors that halving the dose had been the correct course of action. I felt concerned that my blood test results were not reflecting my symptoms of hypothyroidism.

The breathlessness sometimes made me feel as if someone was pressing on my lungs. Due to the exhaustion, I felt as if I was a battery operated doll and that half my batteries had been removed and although the outer shell of me looked roughly the same (apart from becoming increasingly bloated and puffy), I'd lost my functionality.

On half my original dose, I spent the majority of my time lying on the settee. If I attempted to walk outside for a very short distance while holding onto someone, I would drag my feet since I didn't have the energy to lift my feet. Then I would start to have chest pains (which were frightening) and then I would need to sleep for ages. Yet even after sleep, I would never feel refreshed or energised.

I developed balance problems that led to numerous falls. Cognitive difficulties meant that I would mix up the first letters of pairs of words and would find myself using words in the wrong context. I began to think less and less thoughts and found it a struggle to make conversation with others. My sister and I went to see a GP (on emergency) and requested an immediate blood test and also asked to see the NHS specialist as soon as possible (as private patients).

The nausea was extremely unpleasant, it was like being on a ship. When taken on short car journeys, I would retch violently, especially if the car accelerated or went around a roundabout. The pain in various parts of my body was unpleasant.

The wrist and hand pains meant that I was unable to use my hands very much. Simple things such as holding a knife and fork, holding a cup or squeezing the toothpaste tube sometimes hurt so much that I cried with the pain and had to stop what I was doing.

Following the blood test, my sister and I were phoned and told to increase our dose immediately to three quarters of its original level since our TSH levels had at last risen well above normal showing that our dose was too low.

I continued to keep a daily diary and some extracts are shown below;

> *"Nausea & balance problems v. bad. Barely able to walk across room. Nearly fell a few times & felt very sicky. Hands, spine & head also painful. Unable to do anything."*

And

> *"Woke up with carpal tunnel. Nausea and weird feeling in head all morning."*

And

> *"Again virtually paralysed by overwhelming tiredness all day. Needed coat over me as usual even though thermometer showed 26°C."*

After six months taking three quarters of my original daily thyroxine dose, I had not recovered as predicted. I became increasingly concerned that I would never recover on this dose. Only slight improvement occurred and after a further six months on this dose, I remained ill. However, I had been informed that since my blood tests were satisfactory, my thyroxine dose could not be increased further due to the risk to my bones.

My family and friends knew that something was badly wrong especially since my experience was mirrored by my sister's experience. Even strangers knew that something was badly wrong. One day when my mother took my sister and I to the shop, we both attempted to pay for our purchases but the concentration needed to count our change meant that we both fell backwards onto the floor one after the other. From the cashier's sympathetic remarks to our mother, it was obvious that she assumed that we had required ongoing supervision since childhood.

We found a private doctor who was willing to help us and in September 2002 we had our thyroxine dose increased back to its original level, which resulted in some progress. Eventually, we had tri-iodothyronine (T3) gradually included in our treatment with the thyroxine. On first taking T3, I noted that colours seemed brighter and outlines seemed sharper. In addition T3 treatment gave me some intermittent relief from my balance problems but the relief was rationed and mild exertion caused my balance problems to return.

From our mid-twenties onwards, my sister and I developed an increased tendency to worry but assumed that this was an adulthood personality trait. However, my sister and I found that taking T3 gave us temporary relief from the increased tendency to worry. Again the relief was rationed and mild exertion caused this tendency to return. Gradually, my T3 treatment was increased, with every alteration in my treatment came further improvement but my stamina remained abnormally low. I was still rationed in terms of how much I could do each day before I suffered the consequences. If I did too much, old symptoms that I thought had gone would come back.

At the start of 2004, my employers (through no fault of their own) were no longer able to keep my permanent job open until I was well enough to return to work.

Eventually natural desiccated thyroid (NDT) treatment (porcine derived) was included with my T3 treatment and as this natural treatment was increased, my T3 dose was decreased until I was taking NDT treatment (porcine derived) only, which gave rise to further amelioration of my symptoms. My husband told me that my eyes were sparkling since taking this treatment. I felt as if the 'real me' was being rescued.

I felt grateful to my husband, family and friends for their love and support during this difficult experience. I felt very grateful to my private doctor for helping me with my continuing recovery from under treated hypothyroidism. I had no wish to have my NDT treatment (porcine derived) taken away from me due to the devastating consequences that would result from such an action. With the previous few years of my life lost to hypothyroidism, I realised that I was indebted to doctors who were able to treat people like myself.

PART 2

EXPERIENCES OF HYPOTHYROIDISM FROM A SCIENTIFIC STANDPOINT

Preface to Part 2

In part 2, identical twin sisters (C Phillips and D Roach) have described their experiences of hypothyroidism from a scientific standpoint. **Even though they have referred to their own experiences, they have presented part 2 in the third person to increase clarity and brevity.** In addition, they have omitted the emotional, practical and financial implications of hypothyroidism, which are outlined in part 1 of this book.

In chapter 3, 'The evaluation of changes in thyroxine (T4) dose by objective and subjective means in adult identical twin sisters who have been treated for hypothyroidism since childhood' they have illustrated the onset of hypothyroidism during childhood and its treatment with T4. They have also documented the reduction of T4 treatment during adulthood in accordance with blood tests.

A great reliance was placed on blood tests but when their T4 treatment was lowered, they began to develop symptoms of hypothyroidism prior to their blood tests showing that they had become hypothyroid. When their T4 treatment was raised they continued to have ongoing symptoms of hypothyroidism despite their blood tests indicating that they were no longer hypothyroid. The symptoms of hypothyroidism were both severe and diverse. In their case, there was not a consistent correlation between their blood test results and their symptoms of hypothyroidism. They were very concerned at the risks posed to their health by a combination of under reliance on the appraisal of clinical symptoms and over reliance on blood test results.

In chapter 4, 'The evaluation of a thyroxine (T4) dose increase in identical twin sisters with symptoms of hypothyroidism' they have described the reinstatement of the T4 dose that they had taken since childhood. This enabled them to recover from some of their symptoms of hypothyroidism. However the progress appeared to level off, as if the same level of T4 was no longer as effective as it had been originally (prior to the prolonged reduction in their T4 dose).

In chapter 5, 'The evaluation of tri-iodothyronine (T3) inclusion with thyroxine (T4) treatment in identical twin sisters with symptoms of hypothyroidism' they have documented the inclusion of T3 with their T4 treatment. They have shown that this correlated with a decrease in many of their symptoms of hypothyroidism for limited periods of time each day. The beneficial effects of T3 decreased when activity was attempted, meaning that their stamina was still abnormally low.

Chapter 6 is entitled 'The evaluation of increases in tri-iodothyronine (T3) treatment and decreases in thyroxine (T4) treatment in identical twin sisters with symptoms of hypothyroidism'. In this chapter, they have outlined how further increases in T3 and decreases in their T4 treatment correlated with further decreases in the frequency, severity and duration of some of their symptoms of hypothyroidism for variable periods of time each day. They have explained that their stamina was still very low and that their symptoms returned or worsened during or after activity.

In chapter 7 which is entitled 'The evaluation of increases in natural desiccated thyroid (NDT) treatment (porcine derived) and decreases in tri-iodothyronine (T3) treatment in identical twin sisters with symptoms of hypothyroidism', they have revealed how this resulted in further recovery.

CHAPTER 3

MARCH 1969 – SEPTEMBER 2002

THE EVALUATION OF CHANGES IN THYROXINE (T4) DOSE BY OBJECTIVE AND SUBJECTIVE MEANS IN ADULT IDENTICAL TWIN SISTERS WHO HAVE BEEN TREATED FOR HYPOTHYROIDISM SINCE CHILDHOOD

Introduction

Identical twin sisters, D Roach (twin D) and C Phillips (twin C) (who are also the authors of this report) developed hypothyroidism during childhood. Twin D developed hypothyroidism before twin C but both were treated with 200 micrograms (mcg) of thyroxine (T4) daily for nearly twenty five years and both developed normally and had good health (as illustrated by the photographs in this chapter).

When they reached their early thirties, both twins were advised that their T4 dose needed to be reduced from 200mcg daily since the level of thyroid stimulating hormone (TSH) in their blood was suppressed. They were advised of concerns regarding possible links between suppressed TSH levels and reduced bone density. They were informed that when their TSH levels were within the reference range they would be on the correct dose (reference ranges and blood test results are shown in appendix 5).

Gregory A. Brent and P. Reed Larsen have stated that 'Given the potential complications of excessive doses, it is important to educate the patient to the fact that a normal serum TSH concentration is the best goal of T4 treatment' [1]. This is a valid goal if normal TSH levels in a particular individual correlate with the absence of symptoms of hypothyroidism.

Eventually the T4 dose was varied from 200 to 150 to 100 and back to 150 mcg daily in both twins simultaneously as prompted by their individual TSH tests. Objective data was recorded at intervals via the National Health Service (NHS) and included DXA scan results and blood test results for TSH, free T4, free tri-iodothyronine (T3) and total cholesterol levels.

Independently of the NHS (and each other), both twins collected further objective and subjective data, to confirm that their correct T4 dose in adulthood as ascertained by their individual TSH levels would not result in any decline in wellbeing. Objective data was collected at intervals by each twin and included urine N-telopeptide (NTx) levels and urine deoxypyridinoline (Dpd) levels. Further objective data was recorded at intervals (by self-monitoring at home) and included body temperature on waking (via a digital thermometer), approximate timing of ovulation (via a home testing kit) and menstrual cycles. Throughout this time each twin kept a subjective record of wellbeing in the form of a daily diary.

Medical history

MEDICAL HISTORY IN CHILDHOOD

The effect of hypothyroidism in childhood is best illustrated by means of the following photographs. Photographs 1 to 5 (below, opposite and overleaf) show both twins prior to the development of hypothyroidism.

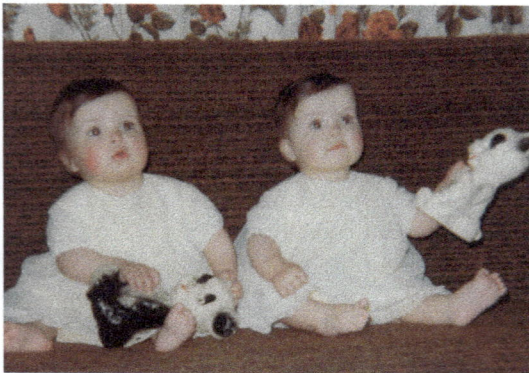

Photograph 1
(taken March 1969, age 1)

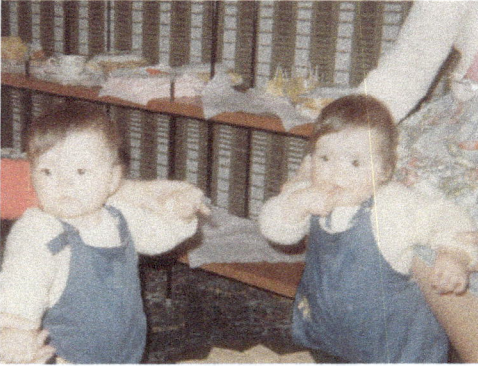

Photograph 2 (taken March 1969, age 1)

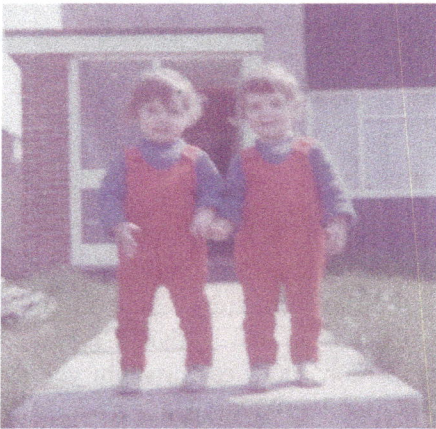

Photograph 3 (taken at age 2)

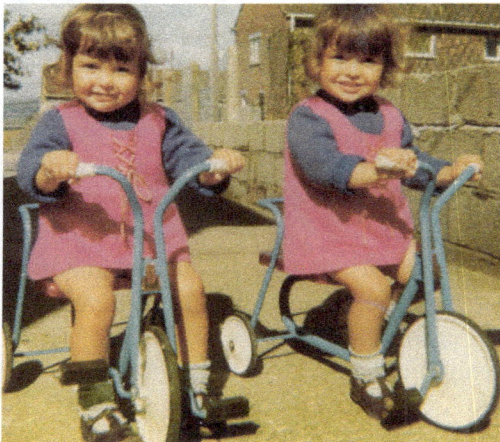

Photograph 4 (taken at approx. age 3)

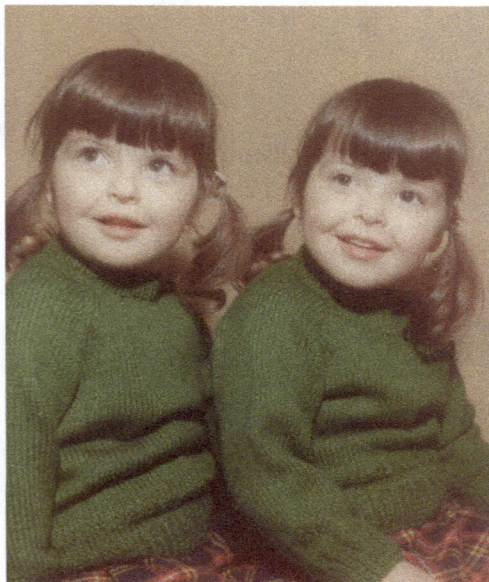

Photograph 5
(taken at approx. age 4)

Photographs 6 and 7 (opposite) show that twin C is still euthyroid and is taller than twin D, who has become hypothyroid. This condition caused twin D to experience stunted growth and development, delayed dental development, weight gain (despite eating the same diet as twin C), severe lack of energy, breathlessness, a dry scalp, some hair loss, a slight yellow pallor to the skin and difficulty with school work. When twin D developed hypothyroidism, it was not recognized by her general practitioners (GPs) whose recommendations were that twin D be put on a low calorie diet and given iron supplements. This did not give rise to any improvement but caused a serious delay in the commencement of appropriate treatment. The twins' dentist queried twin D's delayed dental development, which finally prompted the GPs to enable twin D to see a specialist paediatrician who recognized hypothyroidism immediately and this was subsequently confirmed by tests.

N.B. Photographs 7 and 8 were taken specifically for use in medical lectures given by their specialist paediatrician regarding hypothyroidism in children. They provide incontrovertible medical evidence of the effects of untreated hypothyroidism in childhood.

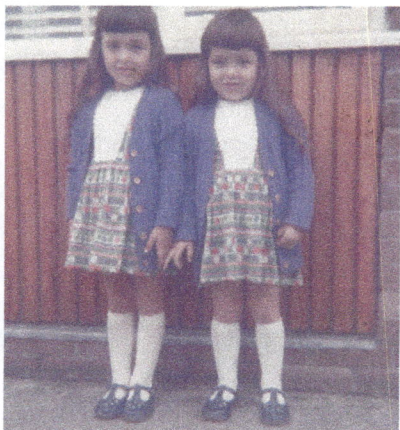

Photograph 6
(taken at age 6)

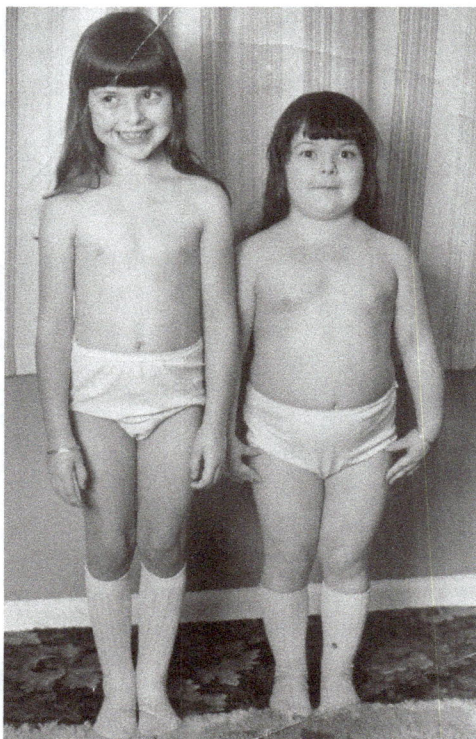

Photograph 7
(taken March 1976, age 8)

Photograph 8 (below) shows that twin C is still euthyroid but twin D has made a dramatic improvement since being treated with T4 and is only slightly shorter than twin C. Twin D's T4 dose was high for a short period and then reduced to 200mcg daily.

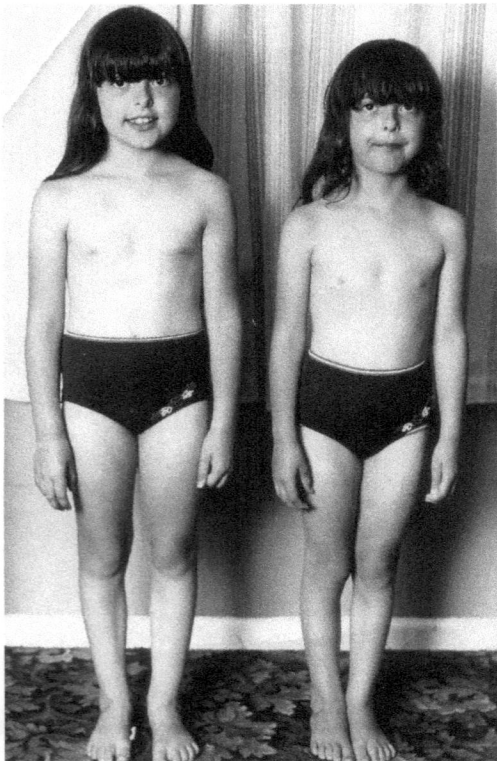

Photograph 8
(taken July 1977, at age 9)

Photograph 9 (opposite) shows that while twin D continues to improve due to the T4 treatment, twin C has become hypothyroid. This condition caused twin C to experience weight gain (despite eating the same diet as twin D), lack of energy and breathlessness. Twin C's hypothyroidism was recognized sooner than had been the case with twin D and treated promptly by comparison. Twin C was treated with 200 mcg of T4 daily.

Photograph 10 (opposite) shows that twin C has recovered from her hypothyroidism since being treated with T4 at 200mcg daily along with twin D. Once again, both twins have similar growth and development.

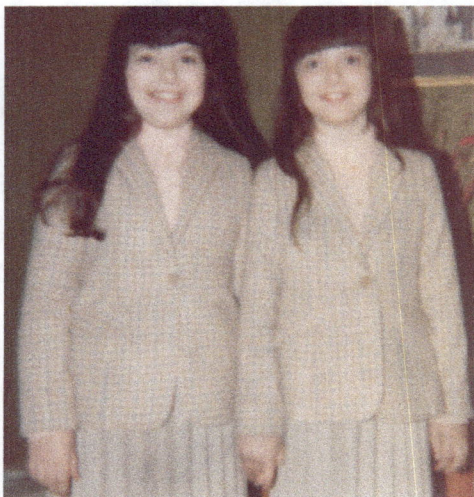

Photograph 9
(taken at approx. age 10)

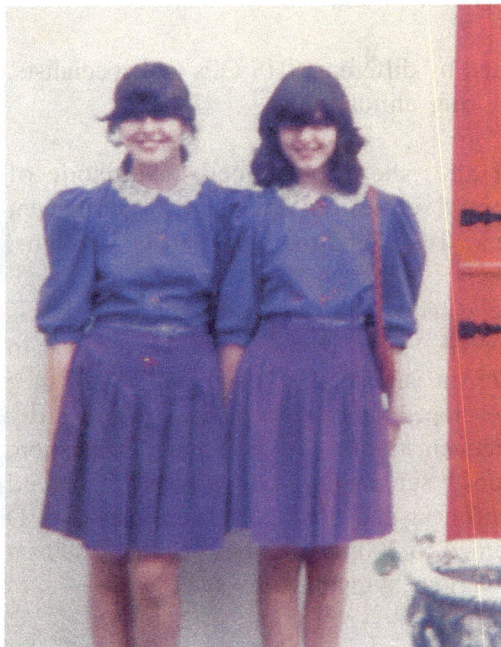

Photograph 10
(taken at approx. age 14)

Photograph 11 (below) shows that due to T4 treatment, the hypothyroidism has not had any apparent detrimental effects in the long term on either of the twins' growth and development.

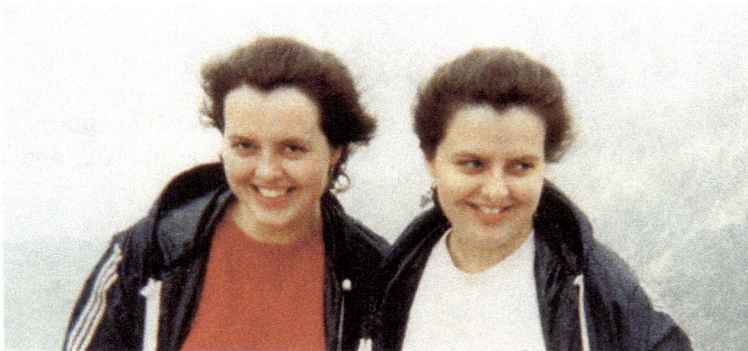

Photograph 11 (taken at approx. age 22)

MEDICAL HISTORY IN ADULTHOOD

In adulthood both twins were treated by different NHS GPs and specialists, to those who had treated them during childhood.

When twin C was 29 years of age, she experienced an episode of labyrinthitis, which caused temporary vertigo but left her with permanent deafness and tinnitus in her right ear. Twin D has no history of labyrinthitis.

When twin D was 31 years of age, a blood test showed undetectable levels of TSH and a raised level of free T4. Twin D was therefore advised to reduce her T4 dose from 200 to 175 (in Summer 1999) and then to 150 mcg daily (in Winter 1999). Twin D developed various symptoms (such as a dry thickened scalp, breathlessness, frequent tingling of the hands, exhaustion, reduced appetite, headaches, cold sensitivity, chest pains, reduced concentration, bloated stomach, puffiness and tinnitus). Therefore, twin D requested that her T4 dose be returned to 200 mcg daily in Spring 2000 (at 32 years of age), after which her various symptoms resolved.

Twin D was later advised that it was clinically impossible for her symptoms to have been due to hypothyroidism due to the fact that her TSH had remained suppressed during this reduction in her dose. No changes were made to twin C's T4 dose at this time.

However, one scientific research study has found that biochemically euthyroid but clinically hypothyroid patients had a favourable clinical response to thyroid replacement, which correlated with the level of thyroid replacement [2].

Another research study later found no support for the hypothesis that people with thyroid function tests within the reference range but symptoms of hypothyroidism benefit from treatment with 100mcg T4 daily [3], however the T4 treatment was not optimised on an individual basis.

DXA scans were subsequently recommended due to concerns regarding the possibility of a link between suppressed TSH and increased risk of premature osteoporosis. When given a DXA wrist scan, twin C's result was normal but twin D's result showed osteopenia. When given a full body DXA scan this demonstrated osteopenia of the hip in both twins. As a result of suppressed TSH levels and the DXA scan results, both twins had their T4 dose reduced from 200 to 150 mcg daily in March 2001 (at age 32). Both twins experienced a sudden onset of symptoms when their T4 treatment was reduced (as shown in Table 1 later in this chapter) which caused a dramatic decline in their wellbeing. A further TSH test prompted a further T4 dose reduction to 100mcg daily in May 2001 in both twins (at age 33), despite their symptoms.

As a result of a further blood test both twins were informed that 100mcg daily was the correct T4 dose for each of them and most symptoms were due to the need for adjustment to the lower dose. At this point, both twins were no longer well enough to continue working.

An increase in the severity of their symptoms led to their request for another blood test that showed that twin C and twin D's TSH levels had risen above the reference range to 16 and 22 respectively. This prompted an immediate and simultaneous increase in their T4 dose to 150mcg daily in September 2001. When TSH levels reached the very lower end of the reference range in both twins, they were each informed that 150 mcg daily was the correct T4 dose and most symptoms were due to the need for recovery after being on a T4 dose of 100 mcg daily.

Following the increase from 100 to 150 mcg of T4 daily in September 2001, some symptoms eventually decreased in frequency and severity (but increased in frequency and severity during or following mild exertion). However, by September 2002 (at age 34), after 12 months on the T4 dose of 150 mcg daily, no further improvement had been noted by either twin for a few months and they were still unable to resume their work and their normal lives. Both twins reported their symptoms and the consequences of their symptoms to their GPs or specialists on a regular basis.

Due to their TSH results, both twins were advised that 150 mcg of T4 daily was the correct dose. It was advised that their T4 dose should not be higher than 150 mcg daily due to the risk to their bones in the longer term.

With regards to ongoing symptoms following the dose reduction below 200 mcg of T4 daily, it was advised that since the TSH levels were satisfactory, not much could be offered from the endocrine point of view.

Advice was requested regarding any possible alternatives to their current T4 treatment.

Objectives

Objective and subjective data was collected on an individual basis in order to personally confirm that the correct T4 dose in adulthood for each twin as ascertained by their TSH levels would not result in a decline in wellbeing.

Method

DXA scans and blood tests for TSH, free T3, free T4 and total cholesterol were carried out by the NHS.

The urine NTx test and the urine Dpd test were carried out by mailing the urine samples to private laboratories. Timing of ovulation was investigated using a home ovulation prediction test.

Waking temperatures were recorded using a digital thermometer, which was placed in the armpit on waking and left for approximately 10 minutes after which time the temperature was recorded.

Menstruation and symptoms were recorded on an individual basis by means of a daily diary. Resting pulse was recorded by twin C only (usually on waking).

Both twins took only the prescribed T4 treatment, therefore subjective observations were not altered by the effects of any other medication. Neither twin has ever smoked.

Results and discussion

Statistical analysis has not been carried out due to the small number of data involved. The objective data was collected on an intermittent basis and is therefore represented as scattered co-ordinates on the graphs.

THE EFFECT OF T4 DOSE CHANGES ON OBJECTIVE CRITERIA MEASURED BY THE NHS (NAMELY TSH, FREE T3, FREE T4, TOTAL CHOLESTEROL AND DXA SCANS)

The thyroid stimulating hormone (TSH) test indicated that the dose of 200mcg of T4 daily was too high in both twins due to an undetectable TSH level. 100mcg of T4 daily was shown to be too low since in both cases it caused the TSH level to rise above the reference range although there was a lag phase before this occurred. However, on 150mcg of T4 daily the TSH appeared at the very lower end of the reference range in both twins. All blood test results and laboratory reference ranges are shown in appendix 5.

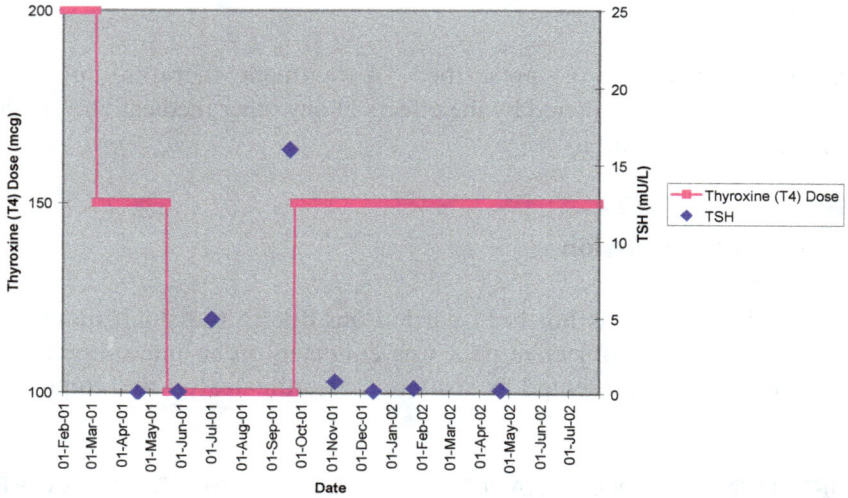

Figure 1. Twin C

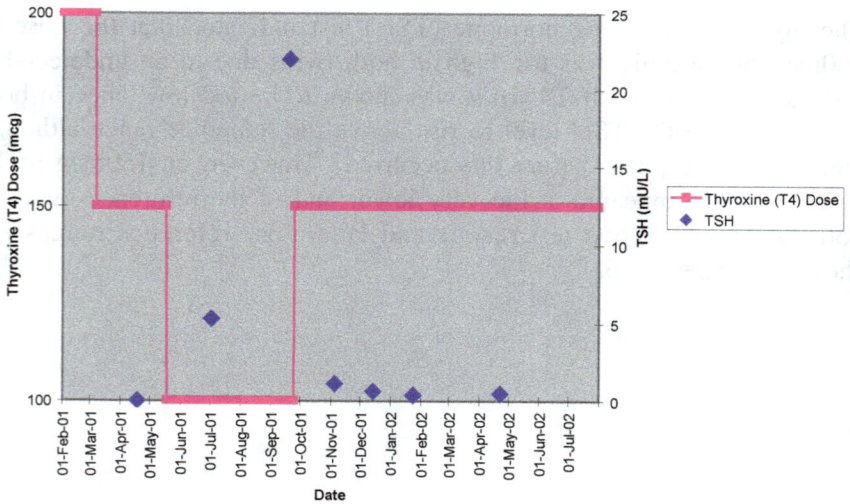

Figure 1. Twin D

Figure 1. The effect of T4 dose on TSH (TSH reference range was 0.35 to 5.00 mU/l at Swansea NHS trust and 0.20 to 4.50 mU/l at Gwent Healthcare NHS trust)

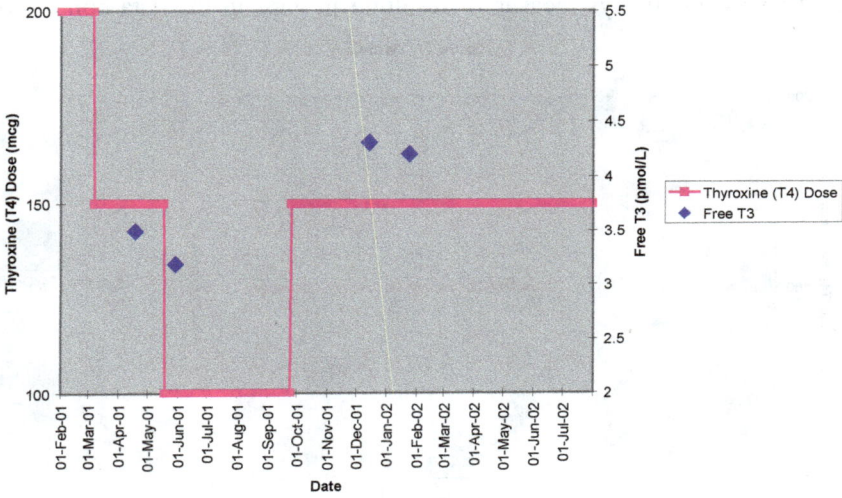

Figure 2. Twin C

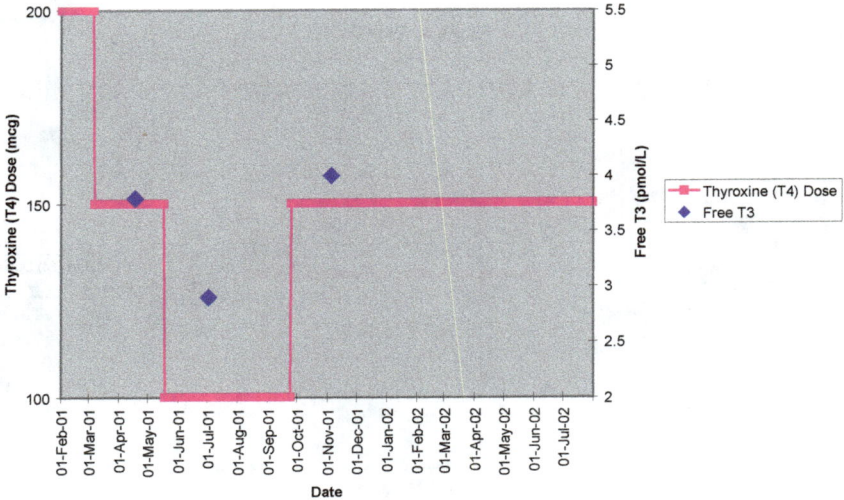

Figure 2. Twin D

Figure 2. The effect of T4 dose on free T3 (Free T3 reference range was up to 5.5 pmol/l at Swansea NHS trust)

Free T3 was lowest at 100 mcg of T4 daily. It was noted that the free T3 reference range at Swansea NHS trust did not include a lower limit and that free T3 was not always measured (resulting in gaps in the data collected).

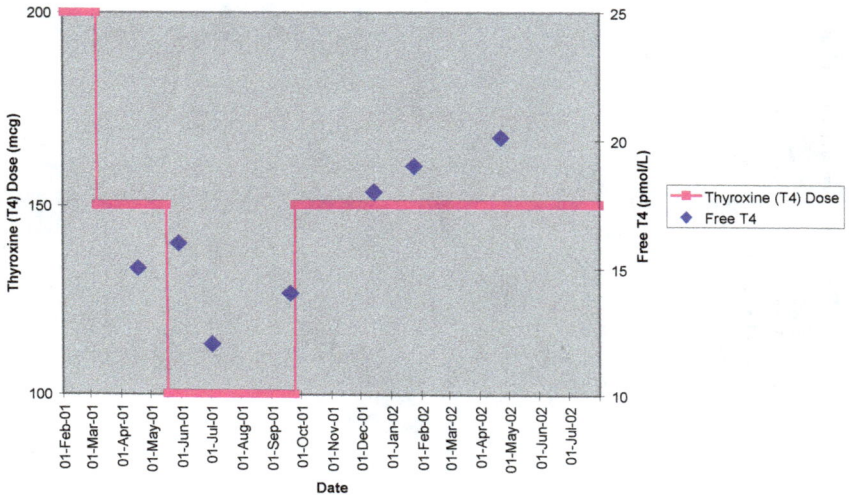

Figure 3. Twin C

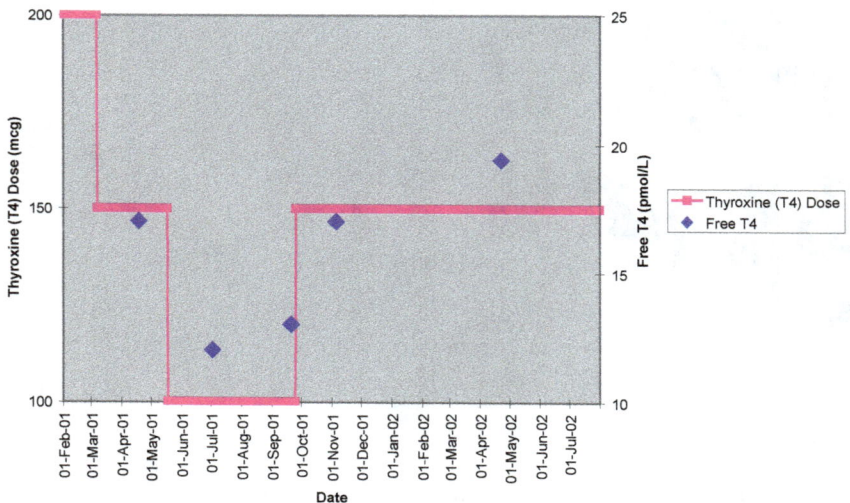

Figure 3. Twin D

Figure 3. The effect of T4 dose on free T4 (Free T4 reference range was 11 to 25 pmol/l at Swansea NHS trust and 10.3 to 24.5 pmol/l at Gwent Healthcare NHS trust)

Free T4 was lowest at 100 mcg of T4 daily. It was noted that free T4 was not always measured.

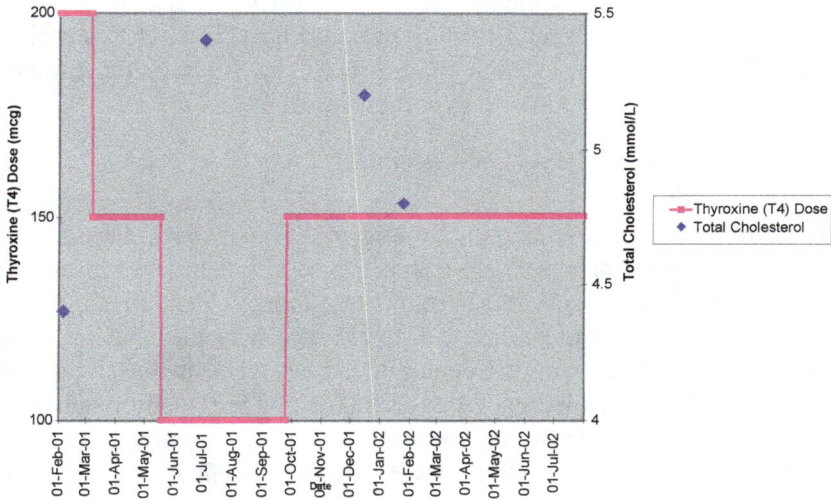

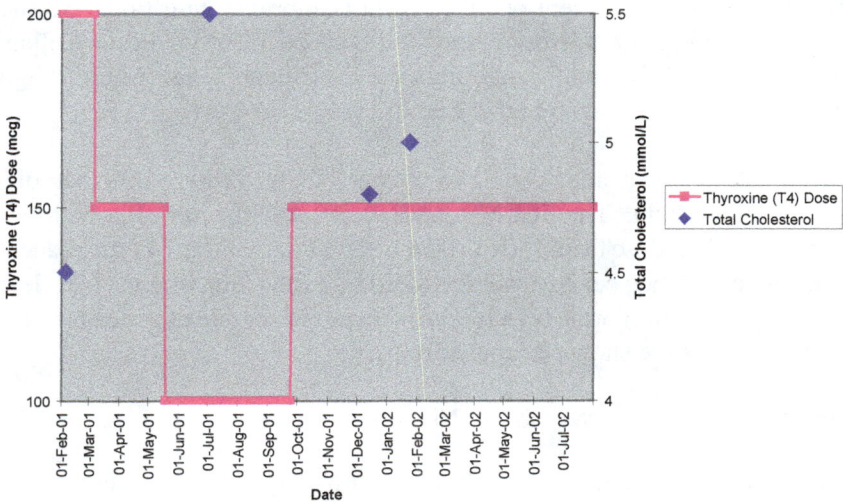

Figure 4. The effect of T4 dose on total cholesterol levels (Total cholesterol normal range was up to 5 mmol/l at Swansea NHS trust)

In both twins, there was an inverse relationship between T4 dose and total cholesterol levels. Total cholesterol was lowest on a dose of 200 mcg of T4 daily and highest and outside the normal range on a dose of 100 mcg of T4 daily. At a dose of 150 mcg of T4 daily, total cholesterol lowered to within the top end of the normal range. Total cholesterol was measured at the request of both twins since it is a parameter known to reflect tissue manifestations of hypothyroidism [4].

THE EFFECT OF T4 DOSE ON DXA SCANS

After nearly twenty five years on a T4 dose of 200 mcg daily, the DXA scan (taken October 2000) for both twins demonstrated osteopenia in the hip (as shown in appendices 1 - 4). After a further 16 months, during which time the T4 dose ranged from 200, to 150, to 100 and back to 150 mcg daily, the DXA scan (taken February 2002) for both twins still demonstrated osteopenia in the hip (as shown in appendices 1 - 4). **However, T4 doses below 200 mcg daily resulted in a marked decrease in activity for both twins, contrary to recommendations that they should increase activity levels for the benefit of bone health.**

THE EFFECT OF T4 DOSE ON NTx LEVELS

The urine NTx results were obtained from Cambridge Nutritional Sciences Ltd. The urine NTx normal range was 0 to 65 in nMol Bone Collagen Equivalents / mMol creatinine at Cambridge Nutritional Sciences Ltd. Higher urine NTx levels indicate a higher rate of bone breakdown.

Unfortunately, it was not possible to obtain NTx readings at 200 mcg of T4 daily for either twin. The first NTx tests were taken the day after both twins had reduced their dose from 150 to 100 mcg of T4 daily. The T4 dose reduction from 150 to 100 mcg per day, was followed by a reduction in urine NTx levels for both twins. Lower urine NTx levels indicate a lower rate of bone breakdown (all NTx results are shown in appendix 6).

THE EFFECT OF T4 DOSE ON URINE DPD LEVELS

(The female normal = less than 7.4 nM Dpd / mM creatinine at BodyWATCH™ International Ltd.)

BodyWATCH™ is the registered trademark of BodyWATCH International Limited.

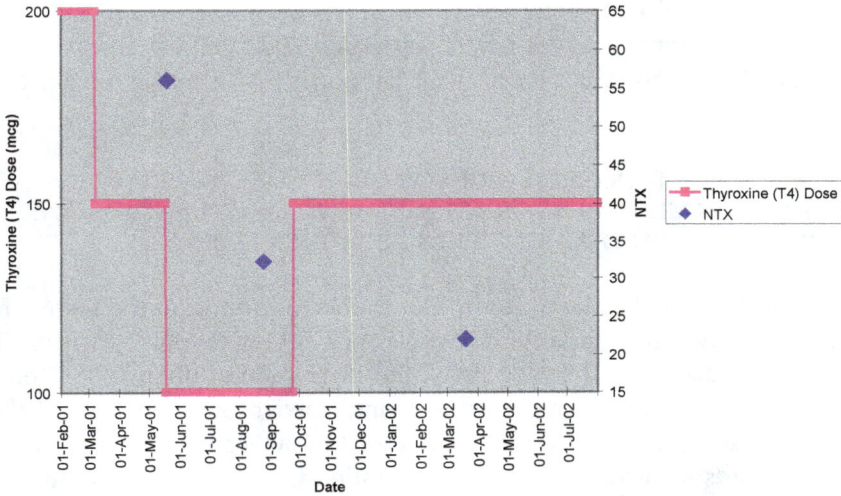

Figure 5. Twin C

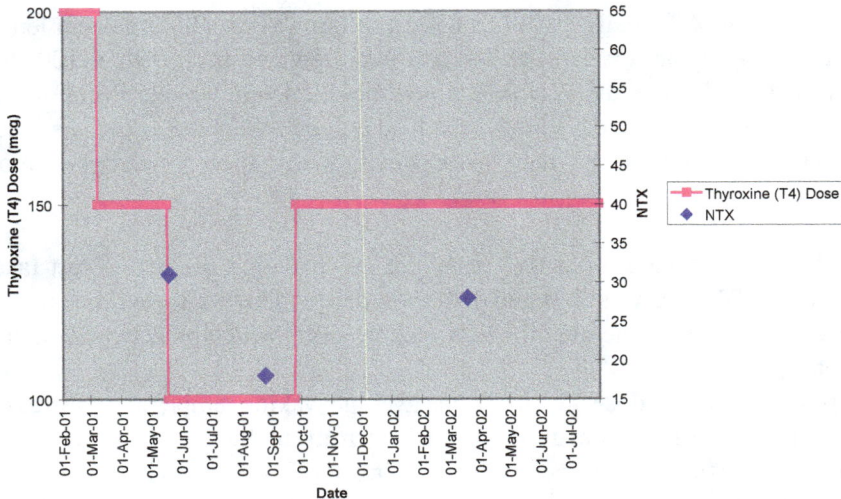

Figure 5. Twin D

Figure 5. The effect of T4 dose on urine NTx levels (The urine NTx normal range was 0 to 65 in nMol Bone Collagen Equivalents / mMol creatinine at Cambridge Nutritional Sciences Ltd.)

Urine Dpd results were obtained from BodyWATCH™ International Ltd. Unfortunately, urine Dpd levels were obtained for both twins only when the T4 dose had been returned to 150 mcg daily. However, since the results were normal (4.3 for twin C in March 2002 and 5.4 for twin D in June 2002) they were consistent with the normal NTx results obtained on this dose.

THE EFFECT OF T4 DOSE CHANGES ON OBJECTIVE CRITERIA MEASURED AT HOME (NAMELY MENSTRUATION, TIMING OF OVULATION, WAKING TEMPERATURE [AND WAKING PULSE FOR TWIN C ONLY])

On 200 mcg of T4 daily, twin C's menstruation usually lasted for approximately 6 days in a 28 day cycle. Twin C noted that when the T4 dose was reduced to 100 mcg daily, the menstruation often lasted for an extra day and was often recorded as being heavier and more painful than usual. When the T4 dose was increased to 150 mcg daily, there was a trend towards menstruation of shorter duration followed by a trend towards menstruation of longer duration but the menstruation was still often recorded as being heavy and more painful.

On 200 mcg of T4 daily, twin D's menstruation was usually 7 days in length in a 28 day cycle. When the T4 dose was reduced to 150 then 100 then returned to 150 mcg daily, twin D noted that the length of menstruation was sometimes one or two days longer than 7 days and was noted as being slightly heavier. In addition, the intervals between menstruation were slightly more erratic.

Both twins obtained a positive result for an ovulation prediction test taken when the T4 dose was 200 and 100 mcg daily. This indicated that neither dose had prevented the luteinizing hormone surge, which precedes ovulation.

In twin D as the T4 dose decreased, the average waking temperature decreased but this was only measured on an intermittent basis. In twin C, the temperature first dipped below 36 °C after the T4 dose had been reduced to 100 mcg daily. The temperature continued to dip below 36 °C intermittently following the increase from 100 back to 150 mcg of T4 daily.

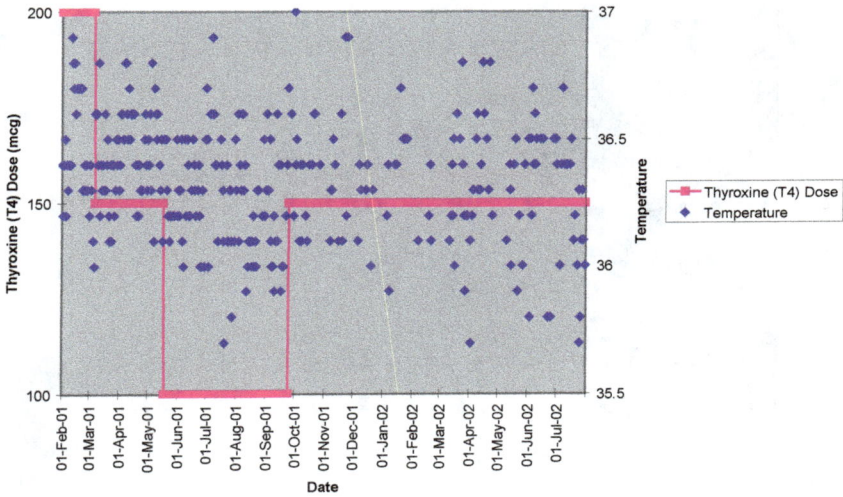

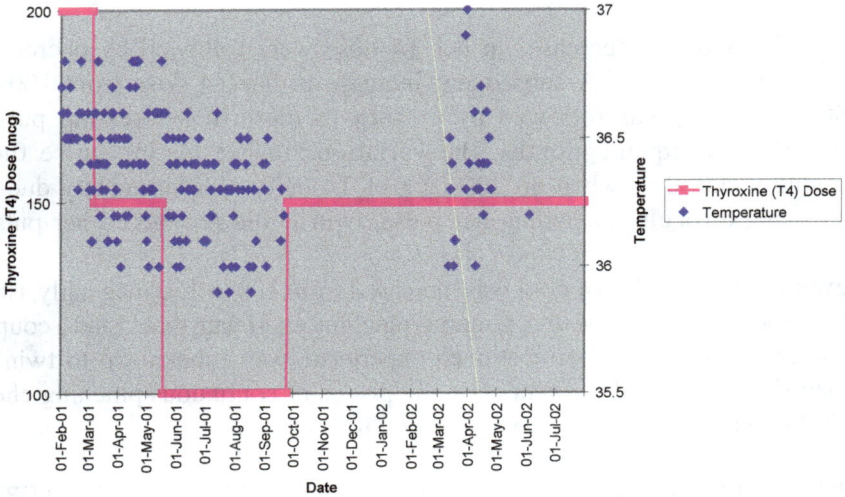

Figure 6. The effect of T4 dose on waking temperature (measured in °C)

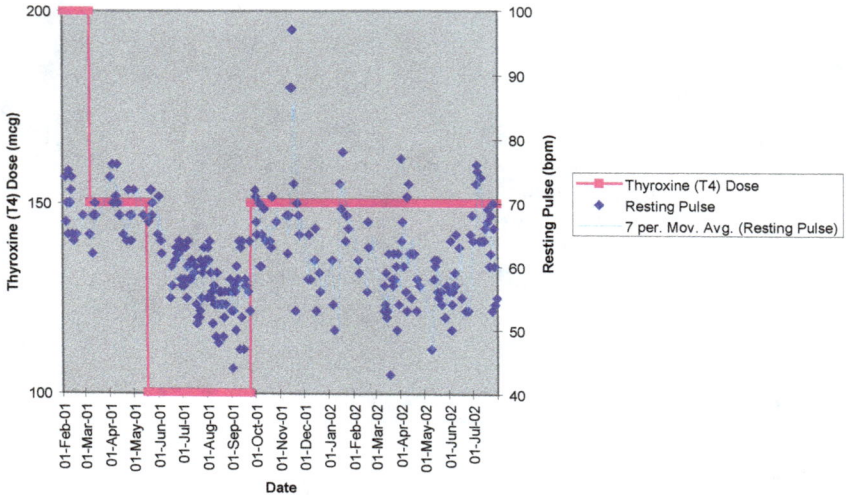

Figure 7. The effect of T4 dose on resting pulse (measured in beats per minute (bpm))

Twin C noted that decreases in her T4 dose were followed by decreases in her resting pulse. A subsequent increase in her T4 dose from 100 to 150 mcg daily, was followed by a sharp increase in her resting pulse. Over the subsequent months, the variations in her resting pulse then became wider, than when on 200 mcg of T4 daily. Unfortunately due to increasing difficulty in finding her pulse, twin D did not record her pulse.

Seven weeks after the T4 dose was increased from 100 to 150 mcg daily, twin D experienced an episode of continuous pinching chest pain that lasted a couple of hours. Twin D's aforementioned experience was unbeknown to twin C when she also started to experience an episode of continuous pinching chest pain that lasted a couple of hours (several hours later).

THE EFFECT OF T4 DOSE CHANGES ON SUBJECTIVE CRITERIA RECORDED AT HOME (NAMELY WELLBEING AS INDICATED BY THE PRESENCE OR ABSENCE OF SYMPTOMS)

On 200 mcg of T4 daily both twins felt well and had no physical symptoms of hypothyroidism. However, when the T4 dose was decreased from 200 to 150 mcg daily, various symptoms developed (as shown in Table 1). When the T4 dose was decreased from 150 to 100 mcg daily, additional symptoms developed and symptoms increased in frequency, severity and duration. When the T4 dose was increased from 100 to 150 mcg daily, symptoms were ongoing and initially additional symptoms continued to develop. Eventually, some symptoms decreased in frequency, severity and duration but continued to have a dramatic impact on the wellbeing and functionality of both twins.

Mild exertion increased symptoms when on 100 and 150 mcg of T4 daily for both twins and resulted in an abnormal increase in sleep requirements. Due to their symptoms both twins were extremely restricted in what they could manage to do each day. In addition both twins noted that their size increased (necessitating the purchase of larger sized clothes since they could not fit into most of their usual clothes). After 12 months on 150 mcg of T4 daily, ongoing symptoms continued to prevent both twins from working and resuming their normal lives.

In this chapter, the effects of T4 dose changes have been documented but the extremely negative impacts of symptoms from an emotional, practical or financial perspective have not been discussed.

Table 1. The effect of T4 dose changes on wellbeing

Sequence of the simultaneous T4 dose changes and the sequence in which the main symptoms subsequently developed.

All the symptoms in italics (whether in bold or not) were experienced by both twins and therefore likely to be due to the T4 dose changes.

The main symptoms still being experienced by each twin when reviewed at the end of August 2002 (after 11 months on 150 mcg of T4 daily) are shown on the following table in bold.

Twin D	Twin C
A. T4 dose reduced from 200 to 150 mcg daily (March 2001)	A. T4 dose reduced from 200 to 150 mcg daily (March 2001)
1. *Dry, thickened scalp (first symptom to develop)*	1. *Dry, thickened scalp (first symptom to develop)*
2. *Breathlessness*	2. *Breathlessness*
3. *Hand, wrist and forearm pain and/ or numbness (causing rationing of hand usage)*	3. *Hand, wrist and forearm pain and/or numbness (causing rationing of hand usage)*
4. *Abnormal exhaustion, low energy (reducing activity)*	4. *Headache, fuzzy head*
5. *Reduced appetite*	5. *Abnormal exhaustion, low energy (reducing activity)*
6. *Headache, fuzzy head*	6. *Bloated stomach, puffiness*
7. *Cold sensitivity (despite adequate room temperatures)*	7. *Cold sensitivity (despite adequate room temperatures)*
8. *Chest pains*	
B. T4 dose reduced from 150 to 100 mcg daily (May 2001)	B. T4 dose reduced from 150 to 100 mcg daily (May 2001)
1. *Inability to work*	1. *Inability to work*
2. *Slowed cognitive function*	2. *Reduced appetite*
3. *Bloated stomach, puffiness*	3. *Chest pains*
4. *Nausea, retching*	4. *Tinnitus (in the ear without pre-existing tinnitus)*
5. *Back pain (mainly spinal)*	5. *Vertigo (visual)*
6. *Tinnitus*	6. *Balance problems (restricting mobility)*
7. *Balance problems (restricting mobility)*	7. *Back pain (mainly spinal)*
	8. *Slowed cognitive function*
	9. *Nausea, retching*
C. T4 dose increased from 100 to 150 mcg daily (September 2001)	C. T4 dose increased from 100 to 150 mcg daily (September 2001)
1. *Visual disturbances (black blobs on periphery of vision)*	1. *Stabbing eye pains and searing head pains*
2. *Stabbing eye pains and searing head pains*	2. *Visual disturbances (black blobs on periphery of vision)*
3. *Coccyx pain*	3. *Coccyx pain*
4. *An episode of continuous pinching chest pain that lasted a couple of hours**	4. *An episode of continuous pinching chest pain that lasted a couple of hours**
5. **Two isolated reddish patches on leg**	5. *An episode of vomiting*
6. *An episode of worsened chest pain*	

* In both twins, the episode of continuous chest pain that lasted a couple of hours occurred 7 weeks after the T4 dose was increased from 100 to 150 mcg daily.

Conclusion

The T4 dose at which both twins had a TSH level appearing within the lower end of the reference range was 150 mcg of T4 daily, but after 12 months on this dose they had ongoing symptoms and reduced wellbeing. This was lower than their original T4 dose of 200 mcg daily at which both twins had been free of physical symptoms, but their TSH levels had been undetectable.

References

[1] Braverman LE, Utiger RD. Werner & Ingbar's *The Thyroid*. Lippincott Williams & Wilkins: 2000. (p. 856-857)

[2] Skinner G R B, Holmes D, Ahmad A, et al. Clinical response to thyroxine sodium in clinically hypothyroid but biochemically euthyroid patients. *J Nutr Environ Med:* 2000 10: 115-124.

[3] Pollock M A, Sturrock A, Marshall K, et al. Thyroxine treatment in patients with symptoms of hypothyroidism but thyroid function tests within the reference range: randomised double blind placebo controlled crossover trial. *BMJ 2001*: 323: 891- 895.

[4] Zulewski H, Muller B, Exer P, et al. Estimation of tissue hypothyroidism by a new clinical score: Evaluation of patients with various grades of hypothyroidism and controls. *JCEM 1997*: 82(3):771-776.

CHAPTER 4

SEPTEMBER 2002 – FEBRUARY 2003

THE EVALUATION OF A THYROXINE (T4) DOSE INCREASE IN IDENTICAL TWIN SISTERS WITH SYMPTOMS OF HYPOTHYROIDISM

Introduction

Identical twin sisters, D Roach (twin D) and C Phillips (twin C) (who are also the authors of this report) developed hypothyroidism during childhood. Both twins were treated with 200 micrograms (mcg) of thyroxine (T4) daily which resolved their symptoms. During adulthood, their blood thyroid stimulating hormone (TSH) levels were suppressed and their dose was reduced to 150 mcg of T4 daily (shortly after this they developed symptoms). Following further blood tests their dose was then reduced to 100 mcg of T4 daily (despite worsening symptoms). Eventually their TSH levels rose above the reference range and their dose was increased to 150 mcg T4 daily.

The T4 dose at which both twins had a TSH level appearing within the lower end of the reference range was 150 mcg of T4 daily but after 12 months on this dose they had many ongoing symptoms, and dramatically reduced wellbeing. Therefore it was necessary for their dose to be returned to 200 mcg of T4 daily during September 2002 and this report has summarized their progress during the 4 ½ months that followed this increase.

Method

Symptoms were recorded on an individual basis by means of a daily diary.

Blood tests for TSH, free tri-iodothyronine (T3), free T4 and total cholesterol were carried out by Swansea NHS trust on 2 January 2003. Urine N-telopeptide (NTx) tests were carried out by mailing urine samples (taken on 4 January

2003 and 8 February 2003) to Cambridge Nutritional Sciences Ltd.

Results and discussion

The effect of a T4 dose increase on wellbeing (as indicated by the presence or absence of symptoms)

Table 1. The main symptoms still being experienced by each twin when reviewed during September 2002 after 12 months on 150 mcg of T4 daily.

Twin D	Twin C
1. Dry thickened scalp	1. Dry thickened scalp
2. Breathlessness	2. Breathlessness
3. Hand, wrist and forearm pain and/ or numbness	3. Hand, wrist and forearm pain and/ or numbness
4. Abnormal exhaustion, low energy	4. Abnormal exhaustion, low energy
5. Reduced appetite	5. Reduced appetite
6. Headache, fuzzy head	6. Headache, fuzzy head
7. Cold sensitivity	7. Cold sensitivity
8. Chest pains	8. Chest pains
9. Bloated stomach, puffiness	9. Bloated stomach, puffiness
10. Nausea, retching	10. Nausea, retching
11. Back pain (mainly spinal)	11. Back pain (mainly spinal)
12. Tinnitus	12. Tinnitus in the ear without pre-existing tinnitus
13. Balance problems	13. Balance problems
14. Coccyx pain	14. Coccyx pain
15. Two isolated reddish patches on leg	15. Vertigo (visual)

Table 2. The main symptoms experienced by each twin during 23 January 2003 after 4 months on an increased dose of 200 mcg of T4 daily (after 4 ½ months no further progress had occurred)

Twin D	Twin C
1. Dry thickened scalp	1. Dry thickened scalp
2. Breathlessness	2. Breathlessness
3. Hand, wrist and forearm pain and/ or numbness	3. Hand, wrist and forearm pain and/ or numbness
4. Abnormal exhaustion, low energy	4. Abnormal exhaustion, low energy
5. Headache, fuzzy head	5. Headache, fuzzy head
6. Bloated stomach, puffiness	6. Bloated stomach, puffiness
7. Balance problems	7. Nausea, retching
	8. Balance problems

In both twins, the increase in the T4 dose from 150 to 200 mcg of T4 daily for 4 months resulted in recovery from some of the symptoms listed in table 1. However, when symptoms were evaluated after a further ½ month on a dose of 200 mcg of T4 daily, no further progress had occurred.

Figure 1. Twin C

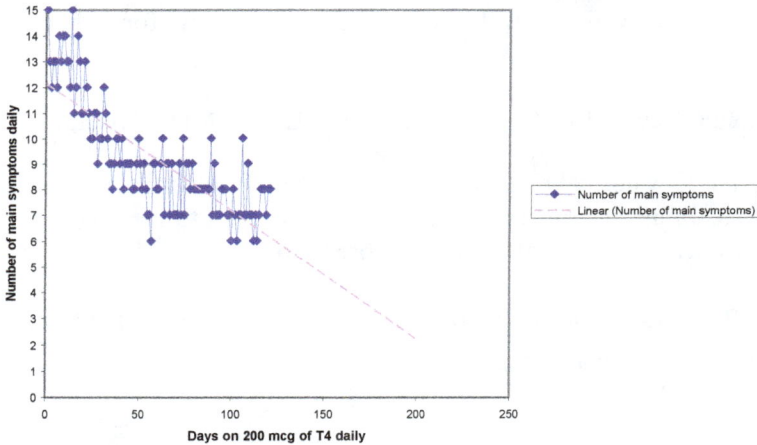

Figure 1. Twin D

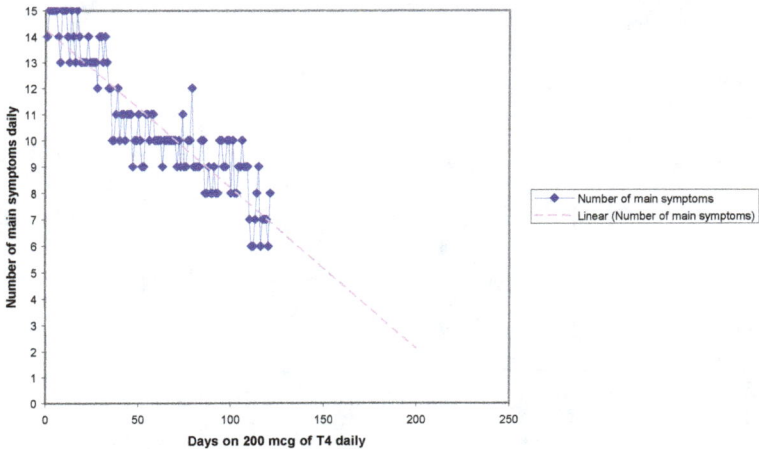

Figure 1. The number of main symptoms (from table 1) experienced each day following an increase in the dose from 150 to 200 mcg of T4 daily (shown for a period of 4 months).

Following an increase in the T4 dose to 200 mcg per day, the number of main symptoms (from table 1) experienced by both twins each day showed a decrease with time during the 4 months represented overleaf. In addition, there was a gradual reduction in the frequency, severity and duration of many of the symptoms experienced each day (although as yet exertion still exacerbated symptoms). After a further ½ month (not represented overleaf), there was no further decrease in symptoms for either twin.

THE EFFECT OF A T4 DOSE INCREASE ON URINE NTX LEVELS

(The urine NTx normal range was 0 to 65 in nMol Bone Collagen Equivalents/ mMol creatinine at Cambridge Nutritional Sciences Ltd.) Higher urine NTx levels indicate higher rates of bone breakdown.

Figure 2 shows previous T4 dose changes and NTx levels for the purposes of comparison.

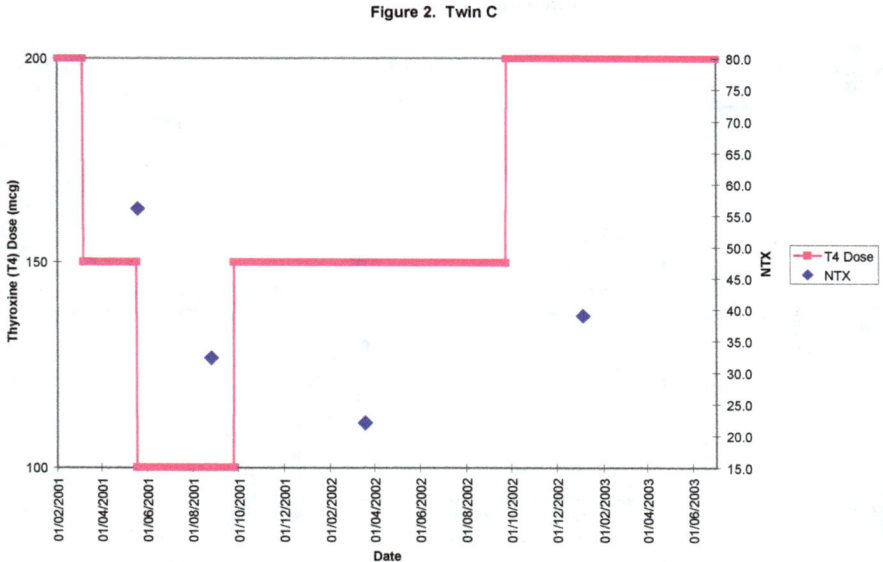

Figure 2. Twin C

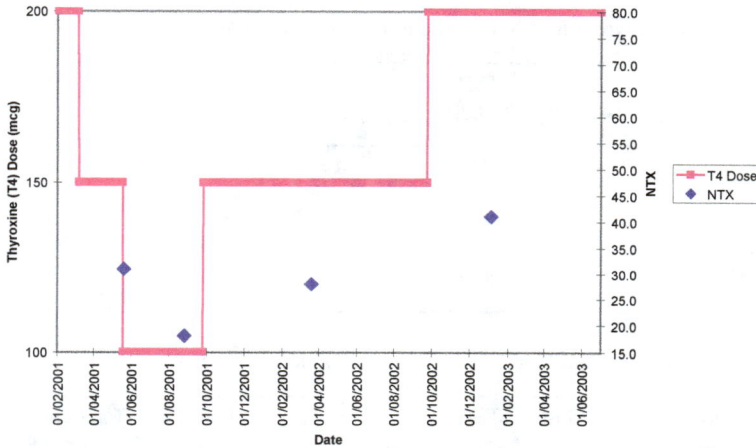

Figure 2. Twin D

Figure 2. The effect of T4 dose changes on urine NTx levels

Figure 2 appeared to show a correlation between T4 dose and subsequent NTx levels.

When the NTx was measured on 8 February 2003 (not represented in figure 2) after 4 ½ months on 200 mcg of T4 only, the NTx values had decreased from 41 to 36 for twin D and from 39 to 32 for twin C. All NTx results are shown in appendix 6.

THE EFFECT OF A T4 DOSE INCREASE ON TSH, FREE T3, FREE T4 AND TOTAL CHOLESTEROL LEVELS

All blood test results and laboratory reference ranges are shown in appendix 5.

On 2 January 2003, the free T4 levels of both twins had risen above the reference range and their TSH levels were undetectable, despite the fact that both twins were still awaiting a reduction in their total cholesterol levels and further recovery from their symptoms. Their free T3 levels were within the reference range.

Table 3. Blood test results for twin D and twin C

D Roach (Twin D) thyroid function (& cholesterol) blood test results

Date	Thyroxine (T4) dose (micrograms daily)	TSH (mU/l)	Free T3 (pmol/l)	Free T4 (pmol/l)	Total cholesterol (mmol/l)
05-Nov-01	150	1.1	4	17	
14-Dec-01	150	0.62			4.8
24-Jan-02	150	0.38			5
22-Apr-02	150	0.46		19.4	
02-Jan-03	200	<0.03	4.2	26.4	5

C Phillips (Twin C) thyroid function (& cholesterol) blood test results

Date	Thyroxine (T4) dose (micrograms daily)	TSH (mU/l)	Free T3 (pmol/l)	Free T4 (pmol/l)	Total cholesterol (mmol/l)
05-Nov-01	150	0.77			
14-Dec-01	150	0.16	4.3	18	5.2
24-Jan-02	150	0.33	4.2	19	4.8
22-Apr-02	150	0.21		20.1	
12-Aug-02	150	0.09	4	21.3	
02-Jan-03	200	<0.03	4.5	28.4	5.1

All blood tests results were provided by Swansea NHS trust except for those taken on 22 April 2002 which were provided by Gwent Healthcare NHS trust.

Conclusion

For both twins, an increase in their T4 dose (to 200 mcg daily) correlated with recovery from some of their symptoms of hypothyroidism.

CHAPTER 5

JANUARY 2003 – JUNE 2003

THE EVALUATION OF TRI-IODOTHYRONINE (T3) INCLUSION WITH THYROXINE (T4) TREATMENT IN IDENTICAL TWIN SISTERS WITH SYMPTOMS OF HYPOTHYROIDISM

Introduction

Identical twin sisters D Roach (twin D) and C Phillips (twin C) (who are also the authors of this report) developed hypothyroidism during childhood. Both twins were treated with 200 micrograms (mcg) of thyroxine (T4) daily. During adulthood, their dose was changed to 150 then 100 then 150 mcg of T4 daily.

After 12 months on 150 mcg T4 daily both twins had a thyroid stimulating hormone (TSH) level appearing within the lower end of the reference range but they had many symptoms of hypothyroidism and dramatically reduced wellbeing. Therefore it was necessary for their dose to be increased to 200 mcg of T4 daily in September 2002 which resulted in a reduction in the number of main symptoms of hypothyroidism experienced each day when evaluated 4 months later. After an additional ½ month, no further improvement was noted.

Therefore between 8 February 2003 and 7 June 2003, the T4 dose of both twins was gradually altered from 200 to 150 mcg daily and simultaneously over the same period their tri-iodothyronine (T3) dose was gradually altered from 0 to 30 mcg daily. It was assumed that T3 was approximately 4 times more potent than T4. This report has evaluated their progress on 8 June 2003, after 4 months with the inclusion of T3 in their treatment.

Method

Both twins started taking T3 on 8 February 2003. Their treatment was divided and taken at intervals through the day.

Blood tests for TSH, free T3, free T4 and total cholesterol were carried out by Swansea NHS trust on 29 May 2003. Symptoms were recorded on an individual basis by means of a daily diary.

Results and discussion

THE EFFECT OF T3 INCLUSION WITH T4 TREATMENT ON WELLBEING (AS INDICATED BY THE PRESENCE OR ABSENCE OF SYMPTOMS)

Table 1. The main symptoms experienced by each twin during 23 January 2003 after 4 months on an increased dose of 200 mcg of T4 daily prior to inclusion of T3 in the treatment

Twin D	Twin C
1. Dry thickened scalp	1. Dry thickened scalp
2. Breathlessness	2. Breathlessness
3. Hand, wrist and forearm pain and/ or numbness	3. Hand, wrist and forearm pain and/ or numbness
4. Abnormal exhaustion, low energy	4. Abnormal exhaustion, low energy
5. Headache, fuzzy head	5. Headache, fuzzy head
6. Bloated stomach, puffiness	6. Bloated stomach, puffiness
7. Balance problems	7. Nausea, retching 8. Balance problems

Table 2. The main symptoms experienced by each twin during 8 June 2003 after 4 months with the inclusion of T3 in their treatment

Twin D	Twin C
1. Dry thickened scalp	1. Dry thickened scalp
2. Breathlessness*	2. Breathlessness*
3. Hand, wrist and forearm pain and/ or numbness	3. Hand, wrist and forearm pain and/ or numbness
4. Abnormal exhaustion, low energy*	4. Abnormal exhaustion, low energy*
5. Bloated stomach, puffiness	5. Bloated stomach, puffiness
6. Nausea*	6. Nausea*
7. Balance problems*	7. Balance problems*

* Symptoms relieved for variable periods of time each day after taking T3

COMMENTS

Both twins noted that the inclusion of T3 in their treatment had a positive effect. However both twins began to experience slight sensitivity to T4 which resulted in slight chest twinges if they took too much T4 in one dose or took T4 without T3.

Certain symptoms namely dry scalp, overall puffiness and hand, wrist and forearm pains were ongoing in both twins despite T3 treatment.

On waking both twins usually had a range of hypothyroidism symptoms (as listed in table 2). However, within half an hour of taking the T3, both twins both found that many of these symptoms (i.e. those marked with * in table 2) were relieved for limited periods of time (depending on activity levels). If they were more restful, the beneficial effects of the T3 lasted for a longer time and vice versa.

In addition, both twins noted a reduced tendency to worry after taking T3. During the parts of the day when symptoms such as balance problems returned, they noted a simultaneous increase in their tendency to worry. They had previously considered this tendency to be an adulthood personality trait that had developed when they were in their mid-twenties and not a symptom of insufficient T3.

When taking T3 for the first time, both twins noted that colours suddenly seemed less dull and the colour red seemed brighter than other colours. After a while, no change in colour brightness was noticed after taking T3 but the colour red still remained brighter than other colours.

THE EFFECT OF T3 INCLUSION WITH T4 TREATMENT ON TSH, FREE T3, FREE T4 AND TOTAL CHOLESTEROL LEVELS

On 29 May 2003, the free T4 levels of both twins had fallen within the reference range but their TSH levels were still undetectable. Their total cholesterol levels had fallen within the normal range. Their free T3 levels were just above the reference range.

Table 3. Blood test results for twin D and twin C

All blood test results and laboratory reference ranges are shown in appendix 5.

D Roach (Twin D) thyroid function (& cholesterol) blood test results

Date	Thyroxine (T4) dose (micrograms daily)	TSH (mU/L)	Free T3 (pmol/L)	Free T4 (pmol/L)	Total cholesterol (mmol/L)
02-Jan-03	200	<0.03	4.2	26.4	5
29-May-03	150 (& 30mcg T3)	<0.03	6.0	17.4	3.9

C Phillips (Twin C) thyroid function (& cholesterol) blood test results

Date	Thyroxine (T4) dose (micrograms daily)	TSH (mU/L)	Free T3 (pmol/L)	Free T4 (pmol/L)	Total cholesterol (mmol/L)
02-Jan-03	200	<0.03	4.5	28.4	5.1
29-May-03	150 (& 30mcg T3)	<0.03	6.3	17.2	4.5

Conclusion

For both twins, inclusion of T3 with their T4 treatment correlated with a decrease in some of their symptoms of hypothyroidism for limited periods of time each day.

CHAPTER 6

JUNE 2003 – MARCH 2004

THE EVALUATION OF INCREASES IN TRI-IODOTHYRONINE (T3) TREATMENT AND DECREASES IN THYROXINE (T4) TREATMENT IN IDENTICAL TWIN SISTERS WITH SYMPTOMS OF HYPOTHYROIDISM

Introduction

Identical twin sisters, D Roach (twin D) and C Phillips (twin C) (who are also the authors of this report) developed hypothyroidism during childhood and were treated with 200 micrograms (mcg) of thyroxine (T4) daily. During adulthood, their dose was changed to 150 then 100 then 150 mcg of T4 daily.

After 12 months on 150 mcg T4 daily both twins had ongoing symptoms of hypothyroidism and it was necessary for their dose to be increased to 200 mcg of T4 daily in September 2002. This resulted in a reduction in the number of symptoms experienced each day when evaluated 4 months later. After an additional ½ month, no further improvement was noted.

Therefore between 8 February 2003 and 7 June 2003, the T4 dose of both twins was gradually altered from 200 to 150 mcg daily and simultaneously over the same period their tri-iodothyronine (T3) dose was gradually altered from 0 to 30 mcg daily. When reviewed on 8 June 2003, inclusion of T3 with their T4 treatment had correlated with a decrease in some of their symptoms of hypothyroidism for limited periods of time each day.

Over a period of 5 months, the T3 dose of both twins was gradually altered from 30 to 90 mcg of T3 daily (and simultaneously during the same 5 months, their T4 dose was altered from 150 to 0 mcg of T4 daily).

In this way their T4 treatment was gradually replaced with T3 between 3 July 2003 and 4 December 2003. It was assumed that T3 was approximately 4 times more potent than T4. Their treatment was divided and taken at intervals throughout the day.

From 4 December 2003 until 12 March 2004 the daily dose of both twins remained at 90 mcg of T3 only. This report has evaluated their progress on 8 March 2004 after 3 months on 90 mcg of T3 only each day.

Method

Symptoms were recorded on an individual basis by means of a daily diary.

Blood tests for thyroid stimulating hormone (TSH), free T3, free T4 and total cholesterol were carried out by Swansea NHS trust on 21 January 2004.

Urine N-telopeptide (NTx) analysis was carried out by Cambridge Nutritional Sciences Ltd for samples collected on 23 September 2003 and 9 March 2004.

Results and discussion

The effect of further increases in T3 and decreases in T4 treatment on wellbeing (as indicated by the presence or absence of symptoms)

Table 1. The main symptoms experienced by each twin during 8 June 2003 after 4 months with the inclusion of T3 in their treatment

Twin D	Twin C
1. Dry thickened scalp	1. Dry thickened scalp
2. Breathlessness*	2. Breathlessness*
3. Hand, wrist and forearm pain and/ or numbness	3. Hand, wrist and forearm pain and/ or numbness
4. Abnormal exhaustion, low energy*	4. Abnormal exhaustion, low energy*
5. Bloated stomach, puffiness	5. Bloated stomach, puffiness
6. Nausea*	6. Nausea*
7. Balance problems*	7. Balance problems*

* Symptoms relieved for variable periods of time each day after taking T3

Table 2. The main symptoms being experienced by each twin on 8 March 2004 after a further 6 months with the inclusion of T3 in their treatment, followed by 3 months on T3 only

Twin D	Twin C
1. Dry thickened scalp	1. Dry thickened scalp
2. Hand, wrist and forearm pain and/ or numbness	2. Breathlessness*
	3. Hand, wrist and forearm pain and/ or numbness
3. Abnormal exhaustion, low energy*	
4. Balance problems*	4. Abnormal exhaustion, low energy*
5. Tinnitus*	5. Bloated stomach, puffiness
	6. Balance problems*

* Symptoms relieved for variable periods of time each day after taking T3

COMMENTS

Due to the onset of intolerance to the synthetic T4, which gave rise to an increased resting pulse, slight chest ache and a burning sensation in the spine shortly after taking the T4, the treatment of both twins was changed to T3 only, in December 2003. Both twins noted that treatment with T3 only, resulted in full relief from all symptoms of intolerance to T4.

Both twins noted that after 3 months on a daily dose of 90 mcg of T3 only, they experienced relief from nausea. Twin D also experienced relief from breathlessness and puffiness.

Treatment with T3 only, had a positive effect and both twins experienced further relief from some of their symptoms for variable periods of the day, however, their stamina was still extremely low and symptoms returned or worsened during or after activity.

Thyroid treatment was always taken on a daily basis. During thyroid treatment changes, treatment was still taken on a daily basis and no gap in thyroid treatment occurred.

THE EFFECT OF T3 (ONLY) TREATMENT ON TSH, FREE T3, FREE T4 AND TOTAL CHOLESTEROL LEVELS

On 21 January 2004, the TSH, free T4 and free T3 were outside the reference ranges. Cholesterol levels had remained within the normal range.

Table 3. Blood test results for twin D and twin C

All blood test results and laboratory reference ranges are shown in appendix 5.

D Roach (Twin D) thyroid function (& cholesterol) blood test results

Date	Thyroxine (T4) dose (micrograms daily)	TSH (mU/l)	Free T3 (pmol/l)	Free T4 (pmol/l)	Total cholesterol (mmol/l)
02-Jan-03	200	<0.03	4.2	26.4	5
29-May-03	150 (& 30mcg T3)	<0.03	6.0	17.4	3.9
21-Jan-04	0 (& 90mcg T3)	<0.03	10.7	<2	3.9

C Phillips (Twin C) thyroid function (& cholesterol) blood test results

Date	Thyroxine (T4) dose (micrograms daily)	TSH (mU/l)	Free T3 (pmol/l)	Free T4 (pmol/l)	Total cholesterol (mmol/l)
02-Jan-03	200	<0.03	4.5	28.4	5.1
29-May-03	150 (& 30mcg T3)	<0.03	6.3	17.2	4.5
21-Jan-04	0 (& 90mcg T3)	<0.03	11.4	<2	3.8

THE EFFECT OF T3 ONLY TREATMENT ON URINE NTX LEVELS

NTx tests were carried out by mailing urine samples to Cambridge Nutritional Sciences Ltd. (The urine NTx normal range was 0 to 65 in nMol Bone Collagen Equivalents / mMol creatinine at Cambridge Nutritional Sciences Ltd.) Higher urine NTx levels indicate higher rates of bone breakdown.

On 23 September 2003 (after 7 ½ months taking both T4 and T3), the NTx levels of both twins had risen just above the normal range to 68 and 69 for twin D and C respectively. When measured again on 9 March 2004 (after just over 3 months taking a daily dose of 90 mcg of T3), their NTx levels had risen further above the normal range to 93 and 79 for twin D and C respectively. All of the NTx results are shown in appendix 6.

Conclusion

For both twins, further increases in T3 correlated with further decreases in the frequency, severity and duration of some of their symptoms of hypothyroidism for variable periods of time each day. However, their stamina remained abnormally low.

CHAPTER 7

MARCH 2004 – SEPTEMBER 2004

THE EVALUATION OF INCREASES IN NATURAL DESICCATED THYROID (NDT: ARMOUR™ THYROID) TREATMENT (PORCINE DERIVED) AND DECREASES IN TRI-IODOTHYRONINE (T3) TREATMENT IN IDENTICAL TWIN SISTERS WITH SYMPTOMS OF HYPOTHYROIDISM

Introduction

Identical twin sisters, D Roach (twin D) and C Phillips (twin C) (who are also the authors of this report) developed hypothyroidism during childhood and were treated with 200 micrograms (mcg) of thyroxine (T4) daily. During adulthood, their dose was changed to 150 then 100 then 150 mcg of T4 daily.

After 12 months on 150 mcg of T4 daily both twins had ongoing symptoms of hypothyroidism and it was necessary for their dose to be increased to 200 mcg of T4 daily in September 2002. Subsequently, it was necessary for their daily treatment to be changed to various combinations of T4 and tri-iodothyronine (T3) and then to T3 only.

From 4 December 2003 until 12 March 2004 the daily dose of both twins remained at 90 mcg of T3 only.

Both twins noted improvements in some of their symptoms for variable periods of time each day but their stamina remained extremely low. Therefore it was necessary to include natural desiccated thyroid (NDT) treatment (porcine derived) (Armour™ Thyroid) in their daily treatment.

For a period of 2 months, their daily NDT treatment (porcine derived) was increased gradually in a stepwise fashion from 0 to 7 x half-grain tablets daily and simultaneously over the same two months their T3 treatment was reduced gradually in a stepwise fashion from 90 mcg to 0 mcg daily. In this way, their T3 treatment was gradually replaced with NDT treatment (porcine derived) from 13 March 2004 to 15 May 2004.

Thyroid treatment was always taken on a daily basis. During thyroid treatment changes, treatment was still taken on a daily basis and no gap in thyroid treatment occurred.

For the following 4 months (15 May 2004 to 15 September 2004) they continued to take 7 x half-grain tablets of NDT treatment (porcine derived) daily. Each half-grain tablet of NDT treatment (porcine derived) was labelled as containing 4.5 mcg of T3 and 19 mcg of T4.

In this report, progress made between 8 March 2004 {prior to taking NDT treatment (porcine derived)} and 15 September 2004 {after 4 months taking 7 x half-grain tablets of NDT treatment (porcine derived) only per day} has been evaluated.

Method

Symptoms were recorded on an individual basis by means of a daily diary.

Blood tests for thyroid stimulating hormone (TSH), free T3, free T4 and total cholesterol were carried out by Swansea NHS trust on 4 June 2004.

Urine N-telopeptide (NTx) analysis was carried out by Cambridge Nutritional Sciences Ltd for samples collected on 25 June 2004, 16 August 2004 and 16 September 2004.

Results and discussion

THE EFFECT OF NDT TREATMENT (PORCINE DERIVED) ON WELLBEING (AS INDICATED BY THE PRESENCE OR ABSENCE OF SYMPTOMS)

Table 1. The main symptoms being experienced by each twin on 8 March 2004 after 3 months on T3 only each day

Twin D	Twin C
1. Dry thickened scalp	1. Dry thickened scalp
2. Hand, wrist and forearm pain and/ or numbness	2. Breathlessness*
3. Abnormal exhaustion, low energy*	3. Hand, wrist and forearm pain and/ or numbness
4. Balance problems*	4. Abnormal exhaustion, low energy*
5. Tinnitus*	5. Bloated stomach, puffiness
	6. Balance problems*

* Symptoms relieved for variable periods of time each day after taking T3

Table 2. The main symptoms being experienced by each twin on 15 September 2004 after 4 months on 7 x half-grain tablets of NDT treatment (porcine derived) only each day

Twin D	Twin C
1. Dry scalp	1. Dry scalp
2. Hand, wrist and forearm pain*	2. Hand, wrist and forearm pain*
3. Exhaustion, low energy*	3. Exhaustion, low energy*
	4. Bloated stomach, puffiness
	5. Balance problems*

*Symptoms relieved for variable periods of time each day after taking NDT treatment (porcine derived)

Comments

Both twins noted that taking 7 x half-grain tablets of NDT treatment (porcine derived) only on a daily basis resulted in further improvement. Twin D experienced relief from tinnitus and twin C experienced relief from breathlessness. Both twins continued to experience balance problems but they occurred less frequently hence on the day that symptoms were evaluated, twin C had balance problems and twin D did not. Both twins had relief from hand pains, exhaustion and balance problems for variable periods of time each day after taking NDT treatment (porcine derived). Both twins also noted an improvement in their stamina after taking this treatment, although their stamina had not yet returned to normal.

THE EFFECT OF NDT TREATMENT (PORCINE DERIVED) ON TSH, FREE T3, FREE T4 AND TOTAL CHOLESTEROL LEVELS

Table 3. Blood test results for twin D and twin C

All blood test results and laboratory reference ranges are shown in appendix 5.

D Roach (Twin D) thyroid function (& cholesterol) blood test results

Date	Thyroxine (T4) dose (micrograms daily)	TSH (mU/l)	Free T3 (pmol/l)	Free T4 (pmol/l)	Total cholesterol (mmol/l)
02-Jan-03	200	<0.03	4.2	26.4	5
29-May-03	150 (& 30mcg T3)	<0.03	6.0	17.4	3.9
21-Jan-04	0 (& 90mcg T3)	<0.03	10.7	<2	3.9
04-Jun-04	7 x half-grains of NDT treatment (porcine)	<0.03	4.9	14.9	4.5

C Phillips (Twin C) thyroid function (& cholesterol) blood test results

Date	Thyroxine (T4) dose (micrograms daily)	TSH (mU/l)	Free T3 (pmol/l)	Free T4 (pmol/l)	Total cholesterol (mmol/l)
02-Jan-03	200	<0.03	4.5	28.4	5.1
29-May-03	150 (& 30mcg T3)	<0.03	6.3	17.2	4.5
21-Jan-04	0 (& 90mcg T3)	<0.03	11.4	<2	3.8
04-Jun-04	7 x half-grains of NDT treatment (porcine)	<0.03	6.3	15.3	4.4

On 4 June 2004, after 3 weeks on a daily dose of 7 x half-grain tablets of NDT treatment (porcine derived) only, the total cholesterol levels of both twins had remained within the normal range. Their free T4 levels had risen to within the reference range. Their free T3 levels had fallen to just above the reference range for twin C and to within the reference range for twin D. The TSH levels of both twins remained below the level of detection.

THE EFFECT OF NDT TREATMENT (PORCINE DERIVED) ON URINE NTX LEVELS

NTx tests were carried out by mailing urine samples to Cambridge Nutritional Sciences Ltd.

(The urine NTx normal range was 0 to 65 in nMol Bone Collagen Equivalents / mMol creatinine at Cambridge Nutritional Sciences Ltd.) Higher urine NTx levels indicate higher rates of bone breakdown. All NTx results are shown in appendix 6.

On 25 June 2004, after 6 weeks on a daily dose of 7 x half-grain tablets of NDT treatment (porcine derived) only, both twins had urine NTx levels, which had fallen to within the normal range. Their NTx levels were 51 and 42 for twin D and C respectively, indicating that they had a normal level of bone breakdown.

On 16 August 2004, twin D's NTx level was 62 and was still within the normal range but twin C had an anomalous reading of 185 which did not correlate with previous results obtained by either twin nor with twin D's current result. A further test result obtained on 16 September 2004 confirmed that twin C's 16 August reading was anomalous.

On 16 September 2004, twin D's NTx level was 61and twin C's NTx level was 36. Although both twins had NTx levels within the normal range, twin D had a higher NTX level than twin C. The reason for this difference was not known since both twins were on the same dose of NDT treatment (porcine derived) and had similar eating patterns. One factor that was no longer the same was their marital status. Although twin C was still married, twin D had divorced in early 2004 (with obvious practical, financial and emotional implications).

Conclusion

After 4 months on a dose of 7 x half-grain tablets of NDT treatment (porcine derived) daily, both twins had experienced further improvements in their recovery and mental wellbeing and were not aware of any adverse effects. In addition, after 4 months on this dose both twins had urine NTx levels within the normal range indicating that they had a normal level of bone breakdown.

Monitoring (via a daily diary recording symptoms and wellbeing) indicated that both twins should remain on NDT treatment (porcine derived) daily (although a slight dose increase still needed to be carried out). In contrast, previous monitoring (via a daily diary) indicated that neither twin should return to treatment with 150 mcg of T4 daily, due to the ongoing symptoms of hypothyroidism that they suffered on this dose (irrespective of satisfactory thyroid function blood test results obtained on this dose for both twins).

On 18 September 2004, both twins had their dose increased to 8 x half-grain tablets of NDT treatment (porcine derived) daily. Both twins extrapolated that this increase in their dose would subsequently lead to recovery from their remaining symptoms and to an increase in their activity levels (which would be of benefit to their bone health).

Both twins hypothesised that 8 x half-grain tablets of NDT treatment (porcine derived) would be the thyroid treatment best suited to their individual needs during adulthood (taking into account both their improving wellbeing and their NTx levels). However they planned to continue to monitor their symptoms to confirm whether further improvements in their wellbeing would occur and to continue to monitor their pulse, their temperature (using a digital thermometer) and their NTx levels.

REFLECTIONS

AUTUMN 2005

Dear Reader,

This book documents our experiences of hypothyroidism during childhood and adulthood but it also describes our quest for wellness. Hypothyroidism during childhood was a very difficult experience but thanks to the provision of appropriate treatment for our hypothyroidism by an exceptional doctor, we were able to have normal mental and physical development.

On looking back at childhood photographs, when one of us was suffering from untreated hypothyroidism and one of us was well, the difference in our appearances was dramatic. However, a solitary photograph of one of us suffering from symptoms of untreated hypothyroidism (in the absence of the unaffected twin for comparison) does not convey the full extent of the negative impact of this condition. Witnessing the dramatic effects of thyroxine (T4) on our growth and development sparked an early interest in the biological sciences.

We have also described the debilitating symptoms of under treated hypothyroidism in adulthood. The diverse symptoms, which can be caused by hypothyroidism have been vividly described by Diana Holmes in her book, 'Tears Behind Closed Doors' [1]. Mary Shomon has also compiled a list of symptoms that can be experienced by patients with hypothyroidism, in her book, 'Living well with hypothyroidism' [2].

The clinical features of hypothyroidism are described excellently by Dr Gordon R B Skinner in 'Diagnosis and Management of Hypothyroidism' [3]. In our experience, there were both similarities and marked differences in the manifestation of hypothyroidism during childhood compared to adulthood. The symptoms of hypothyroidism vary depending on age and stage of development. The signs and symptoms of congenital hypothyroidism are outlined in the book, 'Maternal and Fetal Thyroid Function in Pregnancy' by J.G. Thorpe-Beeston and K.H. Nicolaides [4].

Some improvements in our health occurred when tri-iodothyronine (T3) was included with our thyroxine treatment. We were intrigued by the improvements in mental wellbeing that we experienced after taking T3. Dr Ridha Arem in the book, 'The Thyroid Solution' has provided information about the connection between the thyroid and the mind [5].

Ultimately it was necessary for us to be prescribed with natural desiccated thyroid (NDT) treatment (porcine derived) and we believe that this is the thyroid treatment best suited to our individual needs in adulthood. Thanks to this treatment, we feel as if we are on an upward spiral towards optimal health.

We have written this book about our experiences of hypothyroidism during childhood and adulthood, from a personal perspective and a scientific standpoint. We feel that it is important for further research to be carried out which gives consideration to the patient's perspective. If awareness of the negative impact of undiagnosed or under treated hypothyroidism is raised, then perhaps some good can arise from an otherwise horrendous experience.

After being housebound due to the dreadful symptoms of under treated hypothyroidism, we are relieved to be able to walk into town without assistance, without extreme exhaustion, aches, pains in the chest and balance problems. We really appreciate being able to accept invitations to meet up with family and friends. Although seemingly ordinary, such activities now feel like massive achievements to us. We are thankful that we are regaining our energy.

We feel grateful that we are being prescribed with NDT treatment (porcine derived) in view of the tremendous ongoing improvements in our health, wellbeing and lifestyle. We know that it would be unethical and inhumane, to deprive us of this treatment, as the consequences would be dire. We hope that this book raises awareness of this. This medication is imported from the United States of America, as it is not available in the United Kingdom. The use of NDT treatment (porcine derived) when appropriate is supported in the book, 'Solved: The Riddle of Illness' by Dr Stephen E Langer and James F Scheer [6].

In our case, we knew that we were deteriorating long before the thyroid stimulating hormone (TSH) levels in our blood rose to demonstrate hypothyroidism. There was not a consistent correlation between our TSH level and the presence or absence of symptoms of hypothyroidism. Dr Durrant-Peatfield has highlighted the importance of a full clinical appraisal in the diagnosis of hypothyroidism [7].

We feel that the urine N-telopeptide (NTx) test is a useful monitoring tool and found the parallel variations in our NTx levels following changes in our thyroid treatment of interest. Again this is an area, which warrants further research not just for hypothyroid patients but also for those who have problems with bone health.

We do not know why we both developed hypothyroidism during childhood. Research into the genetic and environmental factors implicated in the onset of hypothyroidism is of importance. Barry Groves in his book, 'Fluoride Drinking Ourselves to Death?' draws attention to the anti-thyroid effect of fluoride [8]. In the book, 'Your Guide to Metabolic Health', Dr Gina Honeyman-Lowe and Dr John C Lowe have reviewed research into many nutritional and environmental factors that have an influence upon metabolic health [9].

It is our hope that others who develop hypothyroidism (whether children or adults) will get a timely diagnosis from the medical profession and prescriptions for the thyroid treatment (most suited to their individual needs).

Best wishes,

C Phillips and D Roach

Bibliography

[1] Holmes D. Tears Behind Closed Doors. Normandi Publishing Ltd: 2002.

[2] Shomon M J. Living well with hypothyroidism. HarperCollins Publishers Inc: 2000.

[3] Skinner G R B. Diagnosis and Management of Hypothyroidism. Louise Lorne Publications: 2003.

[4] Thorpe-Beeston J G, Nicolaides K H. Maternal and Fetal Thyroid Function in Pregnancy. The Parthenon Publishing Group Ltd: 1996.

[5] Arem R. The Thyroid Solution. The Ballantine Publishing Group: 1999.

[6] Langer S E, Scheer J F. Solved: The Riddle of Illness. Keats Publishing: 2000.

[7] Dr Durrant-Peatfield B. The Great Thyroid Scandal and How to Survive it. Barons Down Publishing: 2002.

[8] Groves B. Fluoride Drinking Ourselves to Death? Gill & Macmillan Ltd: 2001.

[9] Dr Honeyman-Lowe G, Dr Lowe J C. Your Guide to Metabolic Health. McDowell Health-Science Books, LLC: 2003.

APPENDICES

Appendix 1 – DXA hip scan results for twin D (October 2000)

D. Roach 24/10/00

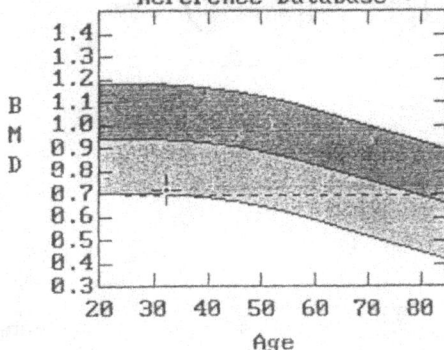

Swansea Osteopc
Q Left Hip
Reference Database •

BMD(Total[L]) = 0.712 g/cm^2

Region	BMD	T		Z	
Neck	0.631	-1.97 74% (25.0)		-1.84	75%
Troch	0.513	-1.88 73% (25.0)		-1.88	73%
Inter	0.826	-1.77 75% (35.0)		-1.74	75%
TOTAL	0.712	-1.89 76% (25.0)		-1.84	76%
Ward's	0.568	-1.42 77% (25.0)		-1.16	81%

• Age and sex matched
T = peak BMD matched
Z = age matched   NHA   02/01/97

Appendix 2 – DXA hip scan results for twin C (October 2000)

C. Phillips 24/10/00

Swansea Osteop

Q Left Hip
Reference Database •

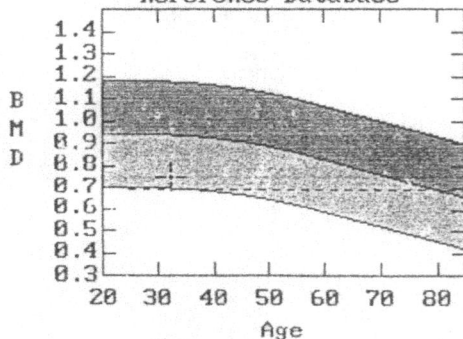

BMD(Total[L]) = 0.743 g/cm^2

Region	BMD	T		Z	
Neck	0.666	−1.65	78%	−1.53	80%
		(25.0)			
Troch	0.545	−1.57	77%	−1.57	77%
		(25.0)			
Inter	0.863	−1.53	78%	−1.51	79%
		(35.0)			
TOTAL	0.743	−1.63	79%	−1.58	79%
		(25.0)			
Ward's	0.552	−1.56	75%	−1.30	78%
		(25.0)			

✦ Age and sex matched
T = peak BMD matched
Z = age matched   NHA   02/01/97

Appendix 3 – DXA hip scan results for twin D (February 2002)

D. Roach 20/02/02

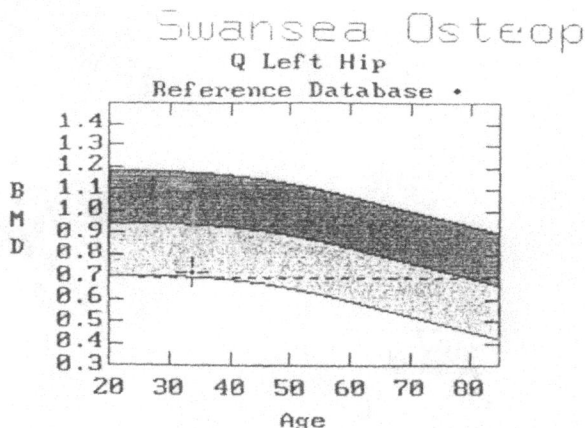

Swansea Osteop
Q Left Hip
Reference Database •

BMD(Total[L]) = 0.712 g/cm^2

Region	BMD	T		Z	
Neck	0.620	−2.06	73%	−1.92	74%
		(25.0)			
Troch	0.506	−1.95	72%	−1.95	72%
		(25.0)			
Inter	0.835	−1.71	76%	−1.70	76%
		(35.0)			
TOTAL	0.712	−1.88	76%	−1.82	76%
		(25.0)			
Ward's	0.567	−1.43	77%	−1.13	81%
		(25.0)			

* Age and sex matched
T = peak BMD matched
Z = age matched   NHA   02/01/97

Appendix 4 – DXA hip scan results for twin C (February 2002)

C. Phillips 20/02/02

Swansea Osteop

Q Left Hip

Reference Database •

BMD(Total[L]) = 0.726 g/cm^2

Region	BMD	T		Z	
Neck	0.627	−2.00 (25.0)	74%	−1.86	75%
Troch	0.508	−1.93 (25.0)	72%	−1.93	72%
Inter	0.859	−1.56 (35.0)	78%	−1.55	78%
TOTAL	0.726	−1.77 (25.0)	77%	−1.71	78%
Ward's	0.574	−1.37 (25.0)	78%	−1.07	82%

◆ Age and sex matched
T = peak BMD matched
Z = age matched   NHA   02/01/97

Appendix 5 – Blood test results for twin D and twin C

D Roach (Twin D) thyroid function (& cholesterol) blood test results

Date	Thyroxine (T4) Dose (micrograms daily)	TSH (mU/l)	Free T3 (pmol/l)	Free T4 (pmol/l)	Total Cholesterol (mmol/l)
20-Jul-99	200	<0.03		30	
18-Oct-99	175	<0.03		20	
21-Jan-00	150	<0.03	4.6	17	
18-Apr-00	150	0.03	3.5	17	
05-Feb-01	200				4.5
18-Apr-01	150	<0.03	3.8	17	
02-Jul-01	100	5.3	2.9	12	5.5
20-Sep-01	100	22		13	
05-Nov-01	150	1.1	4	17	
14-Dec-01	150	0.62			4.8
24-Jan-02	150	0.38			5
22-Apr-02	150	0.46		19.4	
02-Jan-03	200	<0.03	4.2	26.4	5
29-May-03	150 (& 30mcg T3)	<0.03	6.0	17.4	3.9
21-Jan-04	0 (& 90mcg T3)	<0.03	10.7	<2	3.9
04-Jun-04	7 x half-grains of NDT treatment (porcine)	<0.03	4.9	14.9	4.5

C Phillips (Twin C) thyroid function (& cholesterol) blood test results

Date	Thyroxine (T4) Dose (micrograms daily)	TSH (mU/l)	Free T3 (pmol/l)	Free T4 (pmol/l)	Total Cholesterol (mmol/l)
18-Oct-99	200	<0.03		25	
05-Feb-01	200				4.4
18-Apr-01	150	<0.03	3.5	15	
29-May-01	100	0.06	3.2	16	
02-Jul-01	100	4.9		12	5.4*
20-Sep-01	100	16		14	
05-Nov-01	150	0.77			
14-Dec-01	150	0.16	4.3	18	5.2
24-Jan-02	150	0.33	4.2	19	4.8
22-Apr-02	150	0.21		20.1	
12-Aug-02	150	0.09	4	21.3	
02-Jan-03	200	<0.03	4.5	28.4	5.1
29-May-03	150 (& 30mcg T3)	<0.03	6.3	17.2	4.5
21-Jan-04	0 (& 90mcg T3)	<0.03	11.4	<2	3.8
04-Jun-04	7 x half-grains of NDT treatment (porcine)	<0.03	6.3	15.3	4.4

All blood tests results were provided by Swansea NHS trust except for those taken on 22 April 2002 which were provided by Gwent Healthcare NHS trust.

* This result was obtained verbally.

Reference ranges

TSH reference range was 0.35 to 5.00 mU/l at Swansea NHS trust and 0.20 to 4.50 mU/l at Gwent Healthcare NHS trust.

Free T3 reference range was up to 5.5 pmol/l at Swansea NHS trust.

Free T4 reference range was 11 to 25 pmol/l at Swansea NHS trust and 10.3 to 24.5 pmol/l at Gwent Healthcare NHS trust.

Total cholesterol normal range was up to 5 mmol/l at Swansea NHS trust.

Appendix 6 – Urine N-telopeptide (NTx) levels for twin D and twin C

The urine NTx results were obtained from Cambridge Nutritional Sciences Ltd. The urine NTx normal range was 0 to 65 in nMol Bone Collagen Equivalents / mMol creatinine at Cambridge Nutritional Sciences Ltd. Higher urine NTx levels indicate higher rates of bone breakdown.

Date	NTx for twin D	NTx for twin C
19 May 2001	31	56
25 August 2001	18	32.2
19 March 2002	28	22
4 January 2003	41	39
8 February 2003	36	32
23 September 2003	68	69
9 March 2004	93	79
25 June 2004	51	42
16 August 2004	62	185*
16 September 2004	61	36

* This result was anomalous and did not correlate with other results obtained but has been included for completeness only.